STILL SMILING

A Conversation with a Prostate Cancer Survivor

PATRICK WALSH

ISBN: 0991124006
ISBN 13: 9780991124008
Library of Congress Control Number: TXu1-830-864 2013919864
PTW Advisors LLC, Cranford, NJ

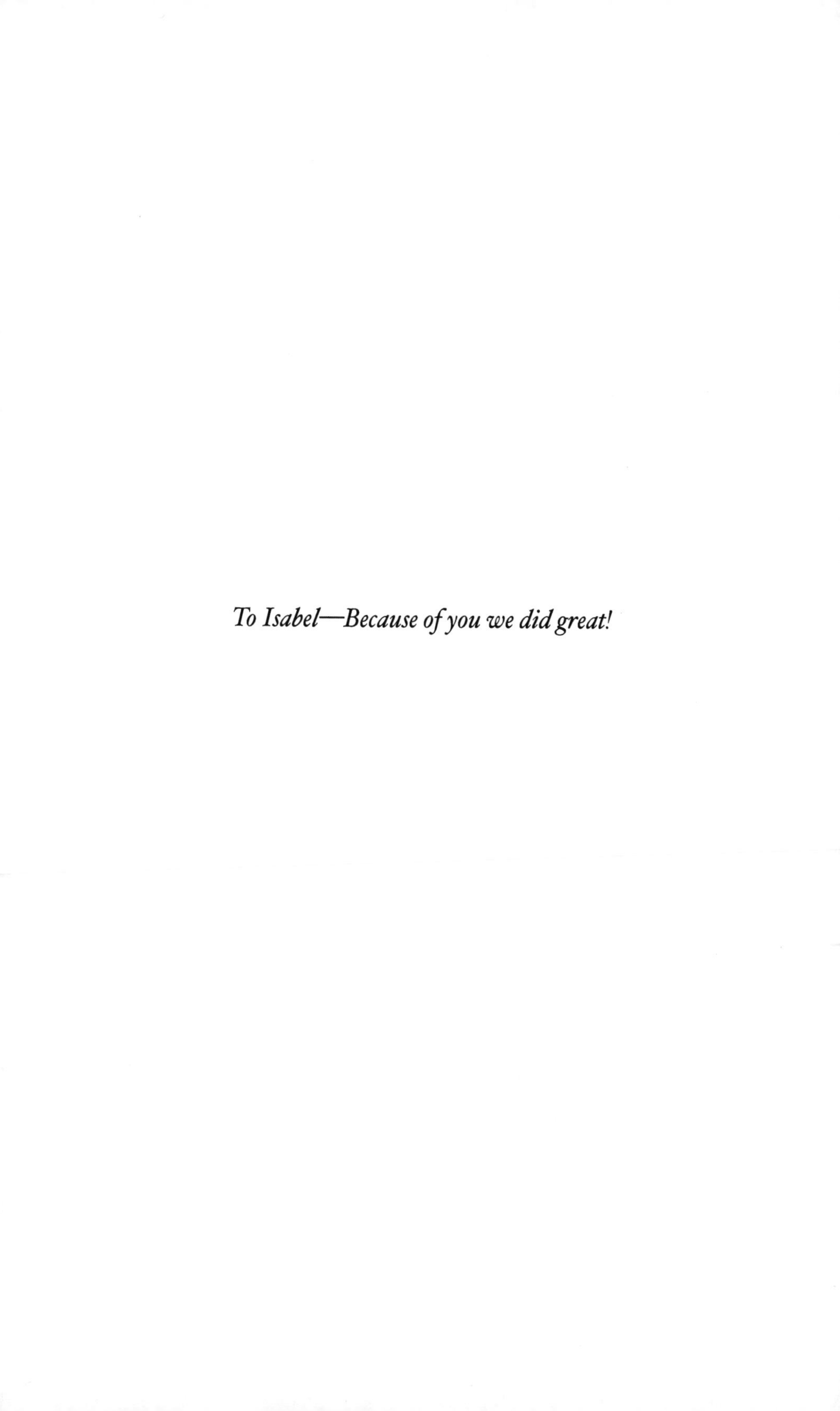

To Isabel—Because of you we did great!

TABLE OF CONTENTS

FOREWORD

When Patrick told me he would be writing a book about his journey, I was elated. I have always been a strong believer in *talking* about cancer, especially prostate cancer. Starting the conversation, in my opinion, has always been half the battle for most men recently diagnosed or facing the possibility of a future diagnosis. Not only has Patrick started the conversation, but he is sharing it with the world after having shared it countless times with other patients of mine.

I remember meeting Patrick and his wife Isabel for the first time in my office. I had seen the expression on his face thousands of times, on thousands of other men going through the same thing. The expression that begs the answers to the questions: "Why me?"—"What now?"—"How much time?"—"Can you help me?"

My answer was simple. "I can help you. You are part of my family now; I will fight for you." I consider all of my patients to be part of my extended family.

Patrick, like many other men in the same position, avoided his cancer. The idea being, if we don't talk about it, if we don't deal with it, then it doesn't exist. But prostate cancer is dubbed "the silent killer" for a reason. One of the most blessed moments in Pat's life was having a urologist who forced him to confront his cancer. As a prostate cancer surgeon, I know firsthand the importance of tackling your disease as soon as possible. Waiting increases the chances of advanced disease and worse outcomes. Unfortunately, many are under the impression that prostate cancer falls under one of two categories: It is an old man's disease; or it is a slow growing disease, so there is no need to treat it. These impressions are myths. Sure, the likelihood of diagnosis is higher in older men, but this does *not* mean that men as young as 40 cannot get prostate cancer *they do*. As far as the trajectory and severity of the disease, it can be slow growing but it can also be aggressive. Each individual case is different, and there is no way to know for sure what the course of the cancer will be. For this reason prostate-specific antigen (PSA) testing is necessary and digital rectal exams (DRE's) are necessary. Prostate biopsies are also necessary when PSA levels are elevated, DRE's are abnormal, and a strong family history of cancer exists.

When prostate cancer is diagnosed, I recommend surgery, specifically robotic surgery. You might ask why I recommend this course of action. Please believe me; it is not just a surgeon trying to do another surgery. I make these recommendations for several reasons, all of which I outlined to Patrick during one of his many visits in my office over the years. Surgery yields quality of life benefits and accurate staging of the cancer's progress. There is this notion that surgery means a lifetime of incontinence and impotence. This is *not* true. Surgery results in the accurate staging of the cancer. Unfortunately, prostate biopsies are random. For example, after PSA testing and a biopsy, your results might indicate that you have a low PSA level and one to three positive biopsy cores. However, you would only know the true nature of your cancer after surgery when your prostate is removed and examined by a pathologist. Hence, the "accurate staging" that surgery provides. After surgery, it is possible to know if you are dealing with cancer that is of a high grade and its level of aggressiveness. Within six weeks after surgery, with PSA monitoring, it is possible to know whether secondary treatment, like radiation, is necessary. As long as your PSA is undetectable, you are cured of this disease. You are in control of your life after surgery.

If you were to choose radiation, you would need to wait at least eighteen months to find out where you stand in terms of cancer staging. America is also getting older and prostate issues associated with old age will still affect those men who opt for radiation. Frequency of urination, incontinence, and other issues associated with enlarged prostate would still be an issue for radiation patients. Surgery, alternatively, would take care of both cancer and future age-related issues.

I have long touted the importance of raising awareness for prostate cancer, and have dedicated my career to the early detection, diagnosis, and treatment of it. Through the development of my own innovative "SMART Technique" (Smart Modified Advanced Robotic Technique), I have been able to ensure the following statistics in my patients: 95 percent prostate cancer cure rate; 96 percent of patients regain continence; 85 percent of patients regain sexual function. There has been no blood transfusion over the last eight years and no major complications. Well, you may say it is too good to be true, but it is true, and here are some of the reasons for this success:

- I have performed close to six thousand robotic surgeries with the da Vinci Prostate Robot.
- I learned as a young urology trainee to be the patient's advocate, to own them and fight to protect them inside and outside of the operating room. There is one thing that I will never negotiate, and I will never let them down: I am the one who performs the *entire* surgery from the beginning to the end and that is very critical to success. If, unfortunately, you or one of your loved ones is diagnosed with prostate cancer, you will want the surgeon you select to perform the surgery. Please do not hesitate to ask him or her if they will perform the surgery or supervise as a trainee performs the surgery.
- During my career as a surgeon I have participated firsthand in the evolution and improvement of prostate surgery from open surgery to laparoscopic surgery to robotic surgery. I can tell you that I have learned many things while participating

> in this evolution. My oncology background and laparoscopic skills from my training in France have contributed greatly to my success rates. The concept is that of three skills or three surgeons in one head.

Always remember when you choose robotic prostate surgery as an option, you are choosing the surgeon behind the technology. I always tell my patients, behind any successful man there is a strong woman and behind any successful robot there is an experienced surgeon. The robot doesn't do the surgery; it is the surgeon and his or her skill.

Frankly, people need both surgical expertise and compassion in order to overcome their disease. I believe strongly in the human aspect of treating prostate cancer, which is the impetus behind having a very carefully selected oncology team to provide care and support for every person.

This is a good time to appreciate what my entire team in the operating room, the anesthesiologist, and my dedicated team in the office do for my patients. Without them I would never be able to stand so strong, and I am truly proud of each and every one of them.

Now back to Patrick Walsh, slightly obese, large volume of cancer, high Gleason score and you would think I would go ahead and take his nerves and surrounding tissue. *No way.* The art of medicine is to remove the cancer while preserving the surrounding nerves responsible for sexual function and continence. Patrick and I formed a strong bond based on his trust and belief in my capabilities and my determination to achieve this trifecta for him. In the end we succeeded!

Support the men you love and make sure that they are knowledgeable regarding prostate cancer and that they are checked annually including a PSA test and a DRE.

I mentioned that I consider all of my patients to be members of my extended family. This is true, yet the heart of my family is my wife Sahar and my beautiful children Jasmine and Alex. Thank you so much for tolerating my lifestyle and allowing me to be there for men like Patrick Walsh twenty-four hours a day, seven days a week.

May God bless you all,

David B. Samadi M.D.

Chairman of Urology at Lenox Hill Hospital

PREFACE

In the fall of 2011, the company I worked for decided it was time to update the pictures of its business leaders on the corporate website, so we all assembled in the lobby of our building to have our pictures taken by a professional photographer. When it was my turn, the photographer stopped in the middle of the shoot and politely asked, "Could you please stop smiling?" He went on to explain that in these types of photographs, you needed to look serious. I complied with his request, but what I wanted to answer was, "No, I *can't* stop smiling. Do you want to know why?" The reason was clear to me: in less than one year, with the help of many wonderful people and a robot, I had overcome denial, fear, and ignorance. I had been diagnosed with and treated for prostate cancer. As I stood there having my picture taken, my life was better than it had been before my diagnosis. So why *not* smile?

There has always been a certain flow to my life. Optimism and joy overcome challenges and setbacks. When I was thirteen years old, my mother died unexpectedly from a pulmonary embolus. Five years later I met my wife, Isabel, and together we built a wonderful family. In my youth I had been a smartass kid who was lucky to get out of high school, but now in adulthood I was the president and chief executive officer of a medical device company that made wonderful life saving devices for people who suffered from heart disease and vascular disease.

I had dedicated the past fifteen years of my professional life to the goals of improving and saving the lives of others, and when the time came for my own life to be saved, I received that same dedication from my urologists, my surgeon, and their teams. I believe this ability to bring joy from sorrow flows from within my soul, and that my soul is an optimistic one!

In December 2010, after being diagnosed with prostate cancer but before my surgery, I decided that I would not let my cancer define my life. What I was really saying was, "My cancer will not defeat me. I will not betray my optimism. I will not become the person who always complains about his health or about having cancer while waiting for the next negative event to occur." I recognized that my story could have been different; without the stern advice of my urologist, I might still be only monitoring my prostate-specific antigen (PSA) levels, burying my head in the sand while my prostate cancer continued to grow, unchecked and untreated, and put my life at risk. Without the skills of my surgeon, I might not have survived my cancer, or I might be living but incontinent and impotent, certainly not enjoying a full and active life. Yet these outcomes did *not* happen, and favorable outcomes like mine are happening every day to other men in similar situations. So I remain optimistic, a cancer survivor, and a believer in optimism and the power of modern medicine.

Although my cancer has not defined my life, it has changed my life. I am much more aware of the value of living every minute of every day. When you are told you have cancer, the finish line can look very close. I could have spent the rest of my time preoccupied with the end, but instead I chose to focus on the remaining journey, no matter its length. I also want my experiences to light the way for other men and their families who may be touched by prostate cancer. I want to share how it felt to be diagnosed with prostate cancer, what robotic surgery and recovery were like, and how my life has changed since the surgery. I want to give them hope that with the proper diagnosis and treatment, there is a good probability that they too will go on to lead happy and productive lives.

My goal is to bring awareness about prostate cancer to as many men as possible. To hell with the idea of the "macho ego"; any topic, if it raises awareness, is acceptable. I admire women and how open they can be about breast and cervical cancer; they discuss them openly and work together toward cures in an organized and public manner. If only more men could act this way regarding prostate cancer. Sure, incontinence and impotence are private topics, but women seem able to move past this privacy issue and enlighten others about detection, diagnosis, and treatments. My wife, Isabel, laughs when she hears me talk to men about gaining control of their urine, getting an erection, and having sex. (Believe me when I tell you that achieving these milestones in that sequence is very important!) She will say to me, "You were so private before you had cancer, but now you talk about anything to anyone." She's right. Up until I was diagnosed with my prostate cancer, I had never spoken to another man, other than my physicians, about prostate-related issues. I wish I had talked to men—men who had had biopsies, men who had had prostate cancer—about their experiences with PSA monitoring, detection, different therapies, their recovery, and life after cancer. If I had, I might have known then what I know now: You can survive prostate cancer and have a wonderful life with both your dignity and your manhood! Such knowledge then would have made my journey much easier to travel.

The idea of writing this book came to me during my recovery. Even though every day continued to be better than the day before, I would find myself asking, why me? I wasn't asking why in a physical sense but in a spiritual sense. I soon realized that maybe I was asking the wrong question; maybe the more appropriate question was "what," as in, "What are you going to do with your experience?" My journey began with ignorance, fear, and denial, but after recovery I was living a healthy and maybe even happier life. Why not tell my story? Not everyone who has or will have prostate cancer will experience the same positive outcome, but at least they would know that there were reasons for hope and optimism. After all, what would life be without hope or optimism? I became even more convinced that this was the right thing to do when my surgeon began referring some of his patients to me so that we could discuss their concerns and my experience with prostate cancer. One thing came through loud and clear from these conversations; this was the first time many of these men had ever discussed prostate cancer with another man. I asked myself why hadn't these conversations taken place, and the only answer I could come up with was that most men are reluctant to speak about something so intimate. The feedback I got from these men was that our conversations were helpful. I thought, *Why not write a book based on these conversations so that any man can read it and in essence have these important and necessary conversations?* One might think the conversation is one sided, given that only I am writing, but my hope is that over time more and more men will speak and share with other men!

I need to state this disclaimer right up front: I am a person, and I was a patient, but I am not a physician. When you read my story, identify with the human elements, understand what it was like to be a patient, and certainly consult with a physician you trust for all medical issues. Please *do not* make medical decisions based on my experience or on the information in this book. If you have not spoken to your physician about prostate cancer, please take the time to speak with him or her and understand this terrible disease and the ways we can beat it!

ACKNOWLEDGMENTS

There are so many people who have given me support during my treatment, recovery, and the writing of this book. But given my story, I have to start with Doctor Tom Giannis, my urologist who forced me to address my cancer and Doctor David Samadi, my surgeon, and his surgical team—You gave me the quality of life I enjoy today. Rosie, thank you for the comfort you gave Isabel and me at a very difficult point in our lives. Helen and Anne, your advice and counsel in my time of need helped me so much, thank you. Tressa, you were my guardian angel in my time of need; words cannot express my gratitude.

To the many men who faced prostate cancer as I did and allowed me to share my story with them, thank you. You helped me recover. I sincerely hope I did the same. Thank you Bob, Gil, John, Renato, Dr. Dennis, Andy, Dr. Frank, David, John, Dr. Mark, Irving, Ron, Mark, Fred, Dr. Phil, Mitch, Mike from Michigan, Nick, Frank, Vince, Glen, and Saul.

Many friends have been with me from the beginning. They shared my sorrow as well as joy, but most importantly they prayed for me! Dr. Luca Lombardi, Carmen and Robert Mosquera, Henry and Sandy Krupinski, Dave and Kathy Berge, Frank and Nancy Cuebelo, Frank and Maria Kozar, Frank and Barbara Kreder, Gary and Becky Hicks, Ron and Ginnie Estel, Harry "Chip" Robinson, Patti Schneider, and Barbara Bator, thank you for giving me so much.

Special thanks to Holly Bosland for supporting me through my entire journey. Holly helped me pick a surgeon, supported me and my family through my recovery, and then edited the many drafts that became this book. Dianna Carthew deserves special thanks.

Dianna was my administrative assistant and confidant when I worked in California. She is one of Isabel's and my dearest friends. Dianna has been with me one might say since I was "in diapers." Her enthusiastic encouragement to write my story was so important to me as I struggled to start the writing process.

Raoul, Philip, and Mike, thank you for helping me find the best surgeon.

Janice Hart, thank you for sharing with me such a personal and inspiring story.

Jim McAvinn, it seems like I have known you forever, and you continue to inspire and encourage me. Thank you for listening, reading my many drafts, and for your suggestions.

Mike Ortega, your calls kept me focused and most of the time on plan. I'm sorry for my many lapses. Mike you are a valued friend; who else would volunteer to take my photo at the risk of breaking their camera?

Dr. Daryoosh Javidi, you are so special to me. Thank you for taking the time to help me focus on my message, my optimism, and most importantly my humanity.

Pat Frustaci, thank you for your friendship; sorry for boring you at our lunches. I know there is much more in the world than prostate cancer awareness and my manuscript.

When I was let go from my job, my former employer generously offered me outplacement services with Meridian Resources. This was a major blessing. Sam Gallucci, thank you for understanding what I wanted to do. Angie Tinnell, thank you for your encouragement as well as help with electronic media and cover design. Mark Richardson, I cannot thank you enough; you mean so much to me but somehow I don't think I have to say anymore than "thank you" for being a wonderful and caring friend who shared his faith and values with me.

My editors at CreateSpace Jennifer G. and Russell thank you for helping me tell my story. Thank you to Jesse Evans at Red 5 Printing in Cornelius, North Carolina you made the cover a reality.

My sister-in-law Rem Gregorio was unfortunately the first of our generation to deal with cancer. Rem you set a high standard for me to emulate.

Damain, Jessica, Sean, and, of course, Nick, thank you for all of your love and support; you are my most valued treasures.

Isabel, thank you for your patience, your patience, and your patience; I love you.

INTRODUCTION TO PROSTATE CANCER

Tag, You're It

"Well, son, you know it's going to get you. It got your father and most of his family." The "son" was me, and the "it" was cancer. Those words, spoken by my dad's third wife, Betsy, just after his death from lung cancer, seemed cruel at the time. In hindsight, however, this wonderful woman was just reminding me of something of which I was already well aware: Cancer is a family affair, and cancer was everywhere in the Walsh family.*

Like the game of tag we play as children, thirteen years later it was my turn. On November 23, 2010, I got the call from one of my urologists: "Mr. Walsh, I am sorry to have to give you this news, but the results of your biopsy came back, and you have prostate cancer." I'm not sure what else he said, but I'm sure it included, "You should make an appointment after Thanksgiving; we need to address this right away." It seems funny now, but my first response to him was, "Thank you for delivering the message in such a caring manner." My wife, Isabel, who was sitting across from me at our kitchen table, actually thought at first that the news was good and that I did not have cancer because I was so calm.

There were to be many emotions over the next year, and I am thankful that calmness and love were some of them. This is the story of my journey.

---

* My father did not have problems with his prostate. This was not a topic we ever discussed, but when I was diagnosed I mentioned to his wife that I could not imagine my father having digital rectal exams or having his PSA monitored. But, to my surprise, she said he had annual physicals and his PSA was consistently around three.

The Prostate Gland, and Prostate Cancer*

The Prostate Gland

The Prostate gland is part of the male anatomy. It is positioned below the bladder and in front of the rectum. The surrounding area also contains many nerve cells and blood vessels that are important to a man's urinary control and his ability to have an erection. A healthy prostate gland will continue to grow until it reaches the approximate size of a walnut. Two important functions of the prostate gland are its role in the male reproductive system and its role in controlling urinary flow. The *reproductive system*—The cells of the prostate gland produce a protein, prostate-specific antigen (PSA), which helps keep semen (the carrier of sperm) liquefied. Some PSA also winds up in the blood stream. The importance of the prostate in the male reproductive system is best stated in the following anecdote. I heard a man ask a urologist the following question, "Doctor, do I need my prostate?" The urologist responded, "Yes, if you want to have children." *Urinary control*—The prostate has muscle fibers, which aid in the control of urine by constricting the urethra, the tube that carries urine from the bladder through the penis (the urethra runs longitudinally, a head to toe orientation, through the center of the prostate). It is not unusual when discussing the urethra passing through the prostate to hear the prostate described as a donut with the urethra passing through the hole of the donut. (See "Very Basic Anatomy")

At some point during my journey it occurred to me that these references to walnuts and donuts had the potential to drive me "nuts" if I let them!

---

* I hope you find this information helpful. If after reading this section you realize you already knew this information, congratulations, you are a lot more knowledgeable than I was when I started my journey. This information was obtained through conversations with physicians and men with prostate cancer as well as from reading literally hundreds of articles on the subject.

Very Basic Anatomy

1. Point of Reference

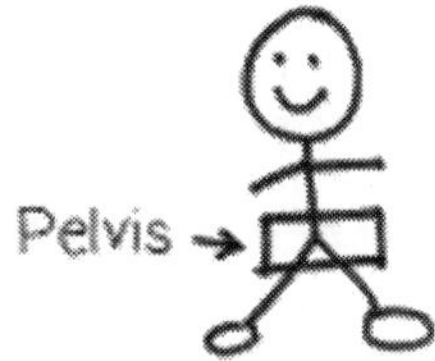

2. Front View of Pelvis

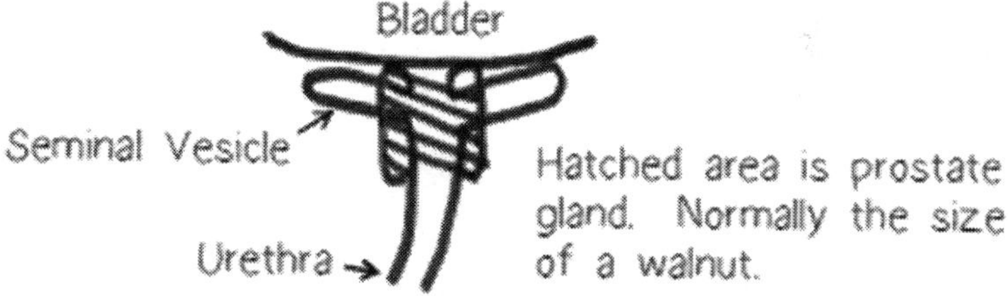

3. Cross section of prostate gland. Sometimes referred to as a doughnut.

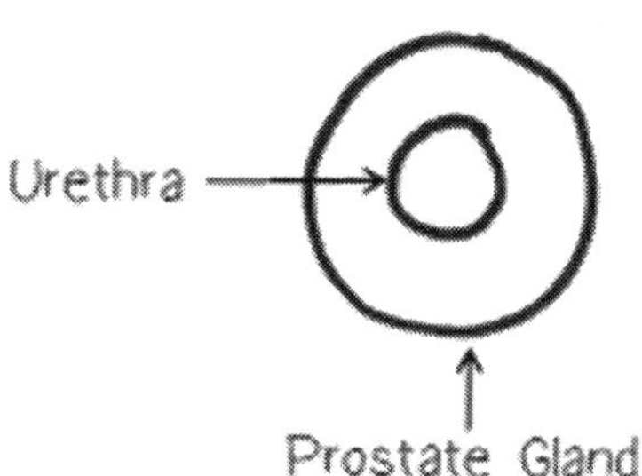

Note: These drawings are rudimentary. They are similar to what we might draw on a napkin or back of an envelope if we were to meet.

Pat
1/21/2014

Prostate Cancer

Prostate cancer starts in the cells of the prostate gland. The cancer cells tend to multiply and form abnormalities that take on a different appearance than healthy prostate cells. One of the most common descriptions of prostate cancer that you will hear is that it is slow growing and that most men will die of something else even though they have prostate cancer. A word of caution about this description: it should not give you a false sense of security that results in you not taking responsibility for your health and reaching out to a physician to better understand prostate cancer. If you have prostate cancer and it begins to grow quickly or spreads to areas other than the prostate, it becomes very dangerous!

Risk Factors[1]

The risk factors for prostate cancer include the following:

- Men over 65.
- Men who eat a high-fat diet, particularly saturated fats.
- Men with a family history of prostate cancer (the risk doubles if a man's father had the disease, and if a brother had it, the risk triples); hereditary prostate cancer typically begins among a cluster of relatives before age 55.
- African-Americans, who have a higher incidence than black men in Africa.
- Possibly, men exposed to such chemicals as cadmium.
- Occupation: rubber industry; cadmium workers.

Symptoms

If you have ever visited a urologist, you may have been asked to fill out a questionnaire prior to meeting with the urologist. More than likely some of the questions were:

- Do you get up to urinate during the night? How many times?
- When urinating do you have a weak stream or difficulty empting your bladder?
- Do you have leakage or dripping after urinating?
- Do you ever have blood in your urine or semen?
- Do you have pain or a burning sensation when you urinate?
- Do you have a slow or inconsistent stream when you urinate?
- Do you experience pain when you have an ejaculation?
- Do you have bone pain or tenderness in the lower back or pelvic area?

One of the reasons you are asked these questions is that they are all signs or symptoms of prostate cancer.[2] The good news is that if you are experiencing any of these symptoms, it does not mean you have prostate cancer, but it does mean you should speak to a physician you trust. Another interesting aspect of these symptoms is that the absence of all or most of the symptoms does not mean you do not have prostate cancer. In fact, many men I have spoken to were like me: they had none of the symptoms yet they were diagnosed with prostate cancer. So, again, what should you do? See a physician you trust, seek an understanding of prostate cancer, have annual physicals, and if something comes up during the physical develop a logical plan with your physician—or you could do as I did (not recommended) live with ignorance and fear.

Methods of Detection

Digital Rectal Exam (DRE) A medical professional inserts a gloved finger into the rectum to feel the prostate for abnormalities, i.e., bumps or hard spots. I found this test relatively painless but somewhat uncomfortable.

Simple Blood Test Blood is drawn and sent to a lab to determine the amount of PSA in the blood. The reliability of this test in detecting prostate cancer is currently being debated. This is probably the biggest debate in the arena of prostate cancer detection. The debate as I understand it centers on the predictive value of the PSA test and the potential to overdiagnose and overtreat prostate cancer. All I can add to this discussion is that I did not have any of the common symptoms of prostate cancer. Without my PSA tests, I might never have been aware that I had a problem until my cancer had spread. This test is painless. I am squeamish about seeing my blood, so I always turn my head.

Needle Biopsy A hollow needle attached to a flexible device is inserted into the rectum. The needle then makes a small perforation in the wall of the rectum behind the prostate and extracts a small core sample of prostate tissue. The number of core samples taken can vary. In my case twelve were taken: six from the left side and six from the right side of the prostate. The core samples are sent to a pathology lab for analysis. A difficult and somewhat painful procedure, the placement of the instrument is uncomfortable and the biopsy instrument made a clicking sound just before taking a sample. I was nervous to begin with, so as the test progressed I became more anxious as I anticipated the click prior to the taking of a sample. After the first few samples I wanted to go home. I know one man who was put to sleep during the process, and he did not feel a thing.

Ultrasound A method of imaging, an instrument is inserted into the rectum. It rubs against the rectal wall behind the prostate.

The goal is to identify abnormalities that the needle biopsy can then target. I did not have this test but I imagine it is similar to the biopsy without the click or needle.

Common Treatments

Active Surveillance also known as Watchful Waiting DREs and blood tests are performed on a regular basis to monitor changes in the prostate or PSA levels. I have also spoken to men who had scheduled biopsies in their surveillance routines. My word of caution is "Don't be like me". Know what you are watchfully waiting for and have a plan if the results indicate a potential problem. I chose watchful waiting and then continued to ignore the results that indicated I had a problem.

Radical Prostatectomy The prostate is surgically removed: *Open*—A surgeon makes a vertical opening below the belly button and removes the prostate through the opening. In some cases the surgeon may make the opening in the perineum, the space between the scrotum and anus, and remove the prostate through the opening. *Laparoscopic*—A surgeon makes several small incisions on the belly. Tools and cameras are then inserted into the incisions. The surgeon performs the prostatectomy through these small incisions. The prostate is physically removed through one of the incisions. *Robotic*—This is the same basic concept as a laparoscopic procedure except that the tools and cameras are connected to a robot that is controlled by the surgeon who is seated at a control console in the operating room.

Radiation therapy A procedure that targets and attempts to destroy cancer cells by exposing them to radiation. There are two types of radiation treatments: *External*—The source of the radiation is outside of the body; a beam of radiation is directed at the targeted cancer cells. *Internal*—Small radioactive seeds are implanted in the prostate targeting the cancer cells. Additionally, if a cancer is aggressive or if initial treatments are not successful, radiation may also be used in combination with chemotherapy and hormone therapy.

This is not meant to be an exhaustive list of treatments. The good news is that as you read this book there are talented people working on new and innovative treatments. When I was diagnosed, a coworker reluctantly approached me. He wanted to respect my privacy, but he felt it would be wrong if he didn't tell me about a device his friend was readying for a clinical trial. The device would attack prostate cancer cryogenically (freezing the cancer cells). Another interesting area of research is focused on understanding the relationship of our genetic makeup as it relates to us being susceptible to diseases like prostate cancer. Hopefully, in the not too distant future, we will be able to determine if our prostate cancer is slow growing and potentially nonlethal or aggressive and lethal by examining our genetic makeup.

Benign Prostatic Hyperplasia (BPH)

This is a noncancerous condition where the prostate continues to grow. When this occurs the urethra may become constricted causing interruptions to or a weak urine flow. Though not cancer this condition needs to be treated by a physician immediately. Treatment may include watchful waiting, change of diet, medication, minimally invasive procedures or surgery.

Facts about Prostate Cancer[3]

- Prostate cancer is the second most frequently diagnosed cancer in American men, following skin cancer.
- It is estimated that one of every seven African-Americans and one in every eight Caucasians develops the disease.

- Although prostate cancer is most common in men over 65, it has been diagnosed in men as young as 40.*
- Prostate cancer is the second most common cause of cancer death in American males and the leading cause of cancer death in males over 85. This high mortality rate may be the result of late detection, since studies show that 87 percent of men treated when their cancer is diagnosed early can expect to be alive in five years.

The Emotions Regarding Prostate Cancer

Each man who will have prostate cancer in his lifetime is loved by someone. He is someone's son, husband, significant other, father, grandfather, friend, or coworker. He is someone you know and love! Because we love these men, we have to make them aware of the seriousness of prostate cancer, screening methods, treatments, and what life can be like after treatment. Some of these discussions may be uncomfortable, but please believe me, they are necessary.

I wish I would have had a conversation about prostate cancer with men who had experienced it. I was monitoring my PSA levels and having digital rectal exams (DREs) annually for ten years, but I never discussed prostate cancer with another man other than my urologist. I never even questioned *why* my internist and urologist were performing DREs! I should have taken my test results more seriously. I thought that if I had prostate cancer, it was slow growing, and I would probably die from something else. In

* Being diagnosed does not mean that you are going to die or even that you will require surgery or radiation treatments. On the contrary, it means that you need to be calm and work with a physician you trust to determine how, based on the facts of your situation, you are going to deal with your cancer. Being diagnosed with prostate cancer is a difficult journey, but if you understand the enemy and the ways you can beat it, your life can be fulfilling and joyful.

the back of my mind, I know I also was afraid of uncomfortable and painful tests, afraid of dying, and afraid of losing my dignity and my manhood! These are real issues that men deal with every day.

IGNORANCE, FEAR, AND DENIAL, THEN REALITY

Ignorance

The first time I heard about PSA was when I got a follow-up letter from my internist regarding my June 30, 2000, comprehensive exam. The form letter from my internist had five sections: an introduction, a list of tests that were normal, a list of tests that were not normal, a recommendations section, and a closing, inviting me to call if I had any questions, as well as a suggested time period for a follow-up physical examination. An asterisk and the letters P-S-A appeared in the "normal" section. There were no numbers, just an asterisk and the three letters P-S-A. I don't recall if I spoke with my internist about this at the time, although if I did it was likely because Isabel would have been after me to call and get some clarity on what PSA was. If I did have such a conversation, I know it did not have an impact on me. I was only fifty-one years old, and other than being overweight, I felt great. My logic told me that if this PSA was a serious issue, it would have merited more than an asterisk and certainly a comment in the recommendations section! Again, to my recollection, this was the first time I had heard about PSA. Imagine that, I was fifty-one!

The next time I heard about PSA was in the follow-up letter to my next comprehensive exam on July 26, 2002. This time the "normal" test section, in addition to the asterisk and the letters P-S-A, showed a number—3.3. The recommendation section again did not contain any reference to PSA or the number 3.3, and I again did not contact my internist to ask what it meant. I didn't want to know.

I think there are a couple of important things to note here about how I regarded my internist's advice and how I managed health issues.

First, in the follow-up letter to my June 26, 2000, physical exam, my internist encouraged me to have another physical in one year. Based on my track record, I evidently thought I knew more than my internist and determined that two years was a better interval. Second, during both physicals I had been given a DRE; I had no idea why he performed that exam or even that the formal name of it was a *digital rectal exam*. (If I had heard of a *digital* rectal exam, chances are I would have thought that it was some kind of binary test, and I suppose I would have been half correct: the finger is either in or out!) Given what I have been through now, I cannot imagine why I never asked my internist *why* he stuck his finger up my rectum each time I had a physical. That was Pat Walsh's "Don't ask; don't tell policy"—I'm too embarrassed to ask, and don't tell me because I don't want to worry. Raising awareness of the need for prostate cancer screening is essential so that other men behave better than me and ask the right questions!

Ignorance Plus Fear

The follow-up letter to my next comprehensive exam on September 28, 2004, identified some changes from my previous physicals. P-S-A no longer appeared in the normal section; it was now in the "tests that were not normal" section. The entry read, "PSA 4.6 (less than 4.5 normal)." The recommendation section now also had an entry: "Any PSA greater than 4.0 should be evaluated. I recommend seeing a urologist."

I first saw a urologist in December 2004. At that visit I had a PSA test and a DRE. My PSA results were 3.3, and the DRE results were normal. The urologist recommended that I have a biopsy of my prostate. I told him I would think about it and went home to do some research on the Internet. I found what I was looking for, but maybe not what I needed. I found articles that spoke about the irrelevance and inaccuracies of PSA screening and the unreliability of prostate biopsies based on the number and origin of biopsy cores. I also learned that a biopsy might result in infection or have the temporary side effect of blood in my semen or stools. I reached out to my internist for advice. I told him that I did not want to have a biopsy because of the potential side effects and that I wanted to continue monitoring my PSA levels. He thought that that was an acceptable strategy, given that prostate cancer is a slow-moving cancer, but he cautioned me that I had to be diligent with regard to PSA monitoring.

Over the next four years, I visited the same urologist eight more times. Each time he checked my PSA level and performed a DRE. The results of the first five PSA tests were in the 3.1–3.8 range ("normal" if I followed the criteria from my internist). Each time, the urologist recommended a biopsy, and I refused, but I was certainly perplexed. The next two PSA test results were 4.2. The DRE results continued to be normal, and I had none of the other symptoms of prostate cancer.

My urologist's advice always remained the same: you should have a biopsy. I always countered with, "No, I want to continue to monitor the situation." In mid-2009 my last PSA test result with this urologist was, I believe, 7.3. I say "believe" because I am not sure I ever followed up with the urologist. He left me a voicemail stating that he was concerned about the results of my PSA test because there had been a dramatic change, and he needed to speak to me.

Why did I ignore his message? Did I hide behind the opinion that I had gotten from the Internet? The answer is yes, but in business,

I never would have accepted that kind of behavior. In my professional role I often said, "Everyone has an opinion; show me data." Why then did I not believe the data the urologist gave me? After all, he did show me probability tables of the occurrences of prostate cancer based on age and PSA level. The answers to my questions are so clear: I was afraid, afraid of CANCER, of what it would do to me and of how it would change my life!

I knew that prostate cancer could rob a man of his dignity, his manhood, and maybe even his life. I thought a prostate cancer survivor's life had to be terrible—certainly worse than my wonderful life. My family life was just starting to settle down. Our children were independent, happy, self-sufficient adults. Sure, they called on us when they needed our support, but that is what family is all about. I was getting ready to enjoy life with the love of my life, Isabel. We enjoyed being around each other and, with our two golden retrievers, we spent weekends at our beach house in Stone Harbor, New Jersey. We also spent part of two years in California. In my professional life, I was the president and chief executive officer of a cardiac surgery and vascular surgery medical device company. My job was meaningful, and I loved it. When I did my job well, I could impact the well-being of patients whose lives were improved by our products while at the same time offering great jobs to the people who designed and manufactured our products. I traveled around the world seeing interesting places and meeting interesting people. Like the t-shirt says, "Life is good!" I ignored the urologist's advice and the data because I was afraid I would lose this wonderful life. Think of how differently I might have reacted if I had spoken to a prostate cancer patient, to someone who had experienced a biopsy, to someone who was a prostate cancer survivor. That is the message of this book: We *have* to talk about prostate cancer—how you can check for it, treat it, and survive it while leading a full and meaningful life!

Ignorance Plus Fear Plus Denial

I knew I had to do something about my PSA level, but I had never returned the urologist's call. Being resourceful, I used insurance as my excuse and went to a new urologist. My logic was simple: the first urologist's group did not accept my insurance, so it was time to move on to another urologist. (It is amazing to me now how I tried to fool myself rather than deal with the issue.) In truth, the urologist's practice had *never* accepted my insurance, *not in the ten years I had been seeing him!* Isabel recommended my new urologist; he had successfully treated her father for bladder cancer many years earlier. I had an appointment with him in September 2010. I brought my ten years of PSA scores with me to the appointment. It went well, but I could sense that he was in charge. His style was friendly but firm and certainly direct. Deep down inside I knew that he was just what I needed. We exchanged pleasantries about our families and our ages, and then he went directly to the point: "Mr. Walsh, we are both the same age. I plan on spending a lot of time enjoying my family and my life. If you plan on doing the same, we need to address your issue." He then performed a DRE, and this time there was no question about why he did the exam. He said my prostate felt normal. I wanted to ask him if he had also checked my eyes for cataracts, but at the time, jokes seemed inappropriate. He instructed me to schedule a blood test in about five days so we could check the status of my PSA. He explained that it was important to wait five days before having the PSA test, because a DRE can cause the prostate to produce more PSA than usual. The wait would allow my PSA levels to go back to my natural level.

After the PSA test in early October, I flew off to Europe for business meetings. I was away for a week, and when I returned on Friday I asked Isabel if the urologist had called. She said, "Yes, you should call him right away." I unpacked my bags, sat alone on the edge of our bed, and made the call. He told me the results; my PSA was 7.3. He explained how serious my situation was and suggested that I have a biopsy right away. I remember telling him that I was still *not* convinced that a biopsy was necessary and that I would continue to monitor my PSA.

I didn't realize it then, but at that moment, he took off the kid gloves and prepared to slap me in the head. In doing so, he was about to save my life. This conversation still lives in my mind, so I am sure I am telling it exactly as it happened.

Urologist: Okay, Mr. Walsh, I understand you want to continue monitoring. I just checked that box on your chart, "patient wants to continue to monitor." You have the right to make this decision. My responsibility is to tell you what you need, and you need a biopsy immediately.

Pat Walsh: Thank you, but I want to continue monitoring my PSA.

Urologist: Okay, Mr. Walsh, can I tell you one more thing?

Pat Walsh: Sure.

Urologist: Mr. Walsh, *you have cancer,* and you will not let me prove it to you. I have seen your file and test results, and I know *you have cancer,* but you will not let me prove it to you. Think about what I have just told you and get back to me on Monday if you change your mind. Have a nice weekend.

Pat Walsh: Not likely.

Call ends.

That call set in motion events that changed everything for me. If he had not been so honest and direct, I would still be fooling myself and running scared while my cancer continued to grow.

Reality

I had the biopsy at my urologist's office on November 19, 2010. Twelve specimens were taken and, believe me, I remember each one. Let's just say this was an uncomfortable procedure. Isabel was in the waiting room. When she saw me after the biopsy she said, "What happened? Your hair is a mess; you don't look good." I asked her to just leave me alone for a few minutes so that I could collect my thoughts. On the way home I did not say much. When we stopped to get coffee, she watched me get out of the car and walk to the coffee shop and said, "You are walking funny!" I laughed out loud and told her, "Of course I am walking funny. It isn't every day that I have a pipe stuck up my ass!" We couldn't stop laughing.

Four days later on November 23, the Tuesday before Thanksgiving, my urologist called with the news—I had cancer. Isabel and I decided that we would not tell the family until after Thanksgiving.

The next day and a half was one of the strangest periods of my life. I know this will sound selfish, but my thoughts were mostly about me and what the world would be like without me. I knew my family was strong and that together they would survive "anything," even if "anything" included my death. I thought about my job—next to my family, there was nothing I loved more. It was noble; the people I worked with cared about each other and our customers. I knew that the business would certainly go on without me. I had many private emotions: Shock, knowing that I really did have cancer. Concern—how bad was my cancer, and had it spread? Sadness—how much time did I have left? Anger over all of the time I had wasted. I tried not to ask, "Why me? Why do I have cancer?" I didn't want to ask, because I truly believed so many good things had happened to me in my life and I had never asked "Why me?" when those had happened, so now I had no right to question why when the bad happened.

A Reason for Joy!

About four in the afternoon of Thanksgiving Day, my life took another turn. We had just arrived at my daughter Jessica's house. Jess and her boyfriend Nick lived in Hoboken, New Jersey. We arrived in two cars; Isabel and I in our car, and my sister-in-law, Rem, and my mother-in-law in Rem's car. Parking on the street in Hoboken is impossible, so the cars needed to be driven to a nearby parking garage. I drove my car, and Nick volunteered to drive Rem's car. While walking back to the apartment from the parking garage, Nick stopped and told me that he wanted to marry Jess. I told him I thought that was a great idea. I knew Jess loved him, and Isabel and I thought he was a great guy, so I was glad he would be part of our family. We agreed that it was our secret and that I would not let Isabel know. Nick planned to surprise Jessica with his marriage proposal while they were on vacation in Arizona. Emotions can change quickly, but now I had a goal; I had to be healthy to walk Jess down the aisle.

Family

Isabel and I had decided to wait until after Thanksgiving to tell the kids about my cancer, so on Sunday, November 28, we called a family meeting at our house. I was as prepared as I was going to be; I would state the facts, talk about potential treatments, and try to reassure the kids that everything would be all right. Damian, our oldest child, and Jess arrived around the same time. Sean, our youngest child, was still in transit from Brooklyn, so we told them to settle down and wait for their brother. Jess sensed that the purpose of this meeting was not good, so she started right in. "What is it? Tell us now. We do not want to wait for Sean!"

That's when it hit me that this was not going to be like the business meetings that I so often ran. Identify the problem, discuss potential solutions, and move forward. This meeting was intensely personal. It was about the love of the people most dear to me, and about my life. My throat started to tighten, my eyes welled, and I knew at that moment this was as intense as love could be—a husband's love for his wife, a father's love for his children, their love reciprocated in full measure, and my love for life.

I am not sure of everything I said, but I know it included, "I have been diagnosed with cancer. It's okay, and everything will be fine." Afterward we all cried together. Jess and Isabel walked around the house. Damian lay on the landing to the steps. I sat in my chair at the kitchen table—the same chair I had sat in for every family meal, the chair I had laughed from, hollered from, and reigned from as coleader of this family. I am not sure how long it was before Sean arrived, but it was obvious to him that there was a major problem. Isabel put her arms around our baby, all six feet, four inches of him, and again I said, "I have been diagnosed with cancer. It's okay, everything will be okay." It wasn't any easier the second time. Again, we all cried.

I always tell people that the most difficult part of my journey was finding out that I had cancer. I still think this is true, because the minute you find out, your life changes. No matter what your priorities are, they change; no matter what you strive for or value, it changes. Mortality becomes extremely real and personal. I had gotten through the previous Tuesday, the day I received my diagnosis, with few or no tears. Facts were facts: I had cancer. Love, however, made this Sunday meeting so much more emotional. It was about our family, about us, about the intensity of our love for each other and for our family—it was about flesh and blood.

We never had another group cry regarding my cancer. I am sure it affected all of us, but it was in our collective nature to persevere and move forward. That night, at 9:41 p.m., I got the following text message from Damian: "Dad, I just want you to know I love you so much. I hope you get better; you mean so much to me. If I could trade places with you, I would in one minute. I really mean that." I replied, "I love you; you are one of my most valuable treasures. I know this will be difficult, but we will pull through this. I am so proud of you. Love, Dad." At that moment, I was sure that with the love of my family and the right surgeon, things would get better!

When I speak to other men who have been diagnosed with prostate cancer, I always think back to that day and ask them if they have family. I remind them how much their family loves them and how important that love will be during their journey.

The Biopsy Results

Isabel and I met with my urologist the week after Thanksgiving. The results of the biopsy indicated that I had a lot of cancer; of the twelve specimens taken, eight had cancer cells. My Gleason score was, I believe, a six. A Gleason score is a subjective, visual (under a microscope), interpretation by a pathologist of the biopsy core samples. The pathologist examines each core sample for the presence of cancer cells. When cancer cells are found, the pattern of the cells are graded from one to five; a one means the cancer cells look similar to normal prostate cells and a five means there is no resemblance to prostate cells. The pathologist does this for the most dominant pattern in the core and again for the second most dominant pattern in the core. The two scores are then added together, the higher the score the more aggressive the cancer is thought to be.

To this day I do not fully understand how the Gleason score is calculated or what it actually represents. I do know that every man I have spoken to who has had a biopsy that resulted in a diagnosis of prostate cancer can tell you his Gleason score. Inevitably he will ask, "What was yours?" I think it is a safe bet that many of them also do not know how it is calculated or evaluated. I mention this because

I believe that for interpretations of things like Gleason scores you need a physician you trust. A lay person newly thrust into the role of cancer patient cannot expect to know all of the nuances of concepts like Gleason scores, let alone make life-changing decisions based on these concepts.

My urologist recommended that I have my prostate removed robotically (a robotic prostatectomy) by a surgeon trained in robotic techniques. He explained that he was a surgeon, but he did not have experience in robotics, and, in his opinion, robotic surgery was the only way to go.* He provided a list of surgeons who performed robotic prostatectomy. He also informed me that I needed a bone scan and CT scans of my abdomen and pelvis to determine whether the cancer had spread.

Computer Tomography CT or CAT SCAN is a diagnostic imaging test that is administered by a technician or a physician who specializes in radiology. Cross-sectional pictures of your body are taken while you lie horizontally on a table that is mechanically moved through the center of the scanner (which resembles a large donut). The benefit over traditional X-rays is that the CT scanner takes many cross-sectional pictures as you move through it. These pictures, when viewed together on a computer monitor, present a three-dimensional image of the area of concern. The scan did not hurt at all. I have heard some people say that it was difficult because they suffer from claustrophobia, but this was not an issue for me. At

* When I am asked why I chose surgery, and specifically a robotic prostatectomy, my answer is simple: My urologist recommended it. I have spoken with other men who have researched various options and can cite the benefits and risks of each, but I didn't do all of that. I simply took my doctor's advice. I don't recommend this approach for everyone, but in my case it worked. I often ask myself why, when I was so reluctant to follow my former urologist's advice regarding a biopsy, I was now willing and preparing to have robotic surgery solely on the recommendation of my new urologist. I wish I had a satisfying answer. Perhaps it was because I now knew I had cancer, and I trusted and needed my urologist to help me beat it. Perhaps it was because I was familiar with robotic surgery from my work with cardiac surgery devices. Ultimately I hope it was the trust I had in my urologist, because I certainly did not have a lot of data or understanding to make this decision on my own.

no time during the scan was my entire body enclosed, given that the scanner was open at both ends and only a few feet wide.

Bone Scan Procedurally my bone scan was very similar to my CT scans except radioactive material was injected into my vein, and I had to wait approximately an hour while the material spread through my body. Based on how the radioactive material shows up in the bones, a physician who specializes in radiology can determine if the cancer has spread to the bones. The scan was of my entire body.

The scans were scheduled for early December,* and events started moving quickly on two tracks. I would be getting my scans at a hospital in New Jersey, and soon I would be working with a team of friends from work on choosing the right surgeon.

The Good News and the Not so Good News

The results of my scans were the first good news we got; the cancer had not spread! The only bad news was that the CT scan revealed I had a kidney stone. Kidney stones are common in my family. My father and my son Damian have had multiple bouts with stones. I have always been cautious about what I ate, based on my father's experience; I limited my intake of hard cheeses, soda, ice tea, and beer, and I tried to drink about a liter and a half of water every day in hopes of avoiding stones. Up until I was sixty years old that strategy worked. But one day in California, I had my first and, until that point only, bout with stones, and it was brutal. When I found out the results of the CT scan, I could not help but wonder what would happen if I passed the stone during or soon after surgery.

* There was something very different about going for the CT and bone scans; it was the first time I entered the hospital as a "cancer patient." The feeling is even today very difficult to describe. I previously had been in this hospital and in the same radiology department when family members required tests, but on this day it was different. The uncertainty that went with my situation caused me to notice and take in everything, yet somehow there was a power that kept all of this from overwhelming me. All I can say is, thank God!

THE RIGHT SURGEON

Research: A Little Help from My Friends

I returned to work the week after Thanksgiving and asked a group of friends and coworkers to meet with me. After explaining that I had cancer and wanted to have robotic surgery, I gave them the list of surgeons my urologist had given me and told them I needed to know which robotic surgeon was getting the best results. Our president of sales responded, "Not a problem. Give me some time; I will have a list of the best surgeons in the area by the end of the day!" The company I worked for develops and manufactures medical devices that support cardiac surgery, and the medical device industry is a small community, so I knew he would use his contacts both inside and outside the company. Three hours later he returned with a short list of surgeons who had performed a significant amount of robotic prostatectomies and gotten outstanding results. There were two surgeons on the top of the list, and the choice was mine.*

Holly, my administrative assistant, took one surgeon from the top of the list, and I took the other, and we sat down at our computers to do some research. I have trusted Holly with my professional life for ten years, and she is one of the main reasons for my success. Isabel and I both know and love Holly and her family. Thus it was

---

* Again my behavior in choosing a surgeon is interesting; in this instance I did not just follow the recommendation of my urologist. I assembled a group of coworkers who I trusted and asked them to help me in my search. Why hadn't I just taken my surgeon's recommendation? His list did not even include the two surgeons that made the list of finalists! Maybe it was my professional experience with cardiac surgery, where the surgeons who perform the most procedures are usually the best, especially with new and emerging technologies. When I look back on my process the only recommendation I would make is, when selecting your surgeon, base your trust in him or her on data. One set of data should show how many procedures they performed and what results they got. I certainly would not want to be the patient of a surgeon who was on the low end of the learning curve.

not an accident that I asked her to help with this important research. I trusted Holly. After I completed my research, I reviewed it with her and asked her opinion. "This guy is God," she replied. "You have to go with him!" I looked at her and continued her analogy, "Holly, in my religion, there are three persons in God—the Father, the Son, and the Holy Spirit. The guy I am researching is one of the other two!" We laughed and exchanged our research. We both recognized that these surgeons were the best of the best, and I trusted that if my cancer could be successfully treated, both surgeons were capable of making that happen. The determining factor, when we finally made our choice, was that only one of the surgeons performed all of the procedures himself. He was the surgeon I wanted.

The choice now made, I asked our president of sales to see if he knew anybody who could get me in for an appointment. Our vice president of marketing knew some personal friends of the surgeon, and soon my appointment was scheduled for early in the morning on December 8.

First Impressions

Isabel and I decided to spend the night of December 7 in New York City. Snow was forecast, and we wanted to ensure we would not miss the appointment. Holly got us a room at the Midtown Marriott and dinner reservations at the Oyster Bar in Grand Central Station. After dinner, we decided to take a walk up Fifth Avenue to look at the holiday decorations. We had taken this walk many times before when we were dating, as young parents, and occasionally when we were out on the town with friends. I thought about all of those times as we walked. Usually we are not a couple who publicly show our affection for one another, but that night we held hands. I thought to myself, so this is what "in sickness and in health, until death do us part" means. Perhaps this was not a deep revelation, but now for the first time we were faced with the possible mortality of one of us. It was just too soon.

My thoughts were about Isabel. We had started dating when I was eighteen and Isabel was seventeen. We were married five years later, and up until this point, our life together had been great. I thought about everything that was happening to her. Her younger sister Rem had been diagnosed with colon cancer earlier in the year, and although Rem was now recuperating, the cancer had taken a toll on her, which worried Isabel. Over the summer, our daughter Jess had been in a bicycle accident while competing in a triathlon, and even with a helmet, she had fractured her skull in two places. Jess also was recovering, but her condition concerned us both (remember too that Isabel was not yet aware that Nick was going to ask Jess to marry him). Now, on top of all of that, Isabel was getting ready to see a surgeon about my own cancer.

We returned to the hotel, and after a good night's sleep we headed uptown for our appointment with the surgeon. A light dusting of snow covered the ground. The office we were headed for was in a wonderful neighborhood of nice shops, so the walk was pleasant even though our thoughts were serious. As we entered the building, I wondered about the surgeon himself. In my job, I had been exposed to many world-famous cardiac surgeons. Whereas most were down to earth, pleasant, and approachable, others thought of themselves as gods who should be treated as such. I wondered which type of surgeon ours would be.

We were early for our appointment. The public area of the office was open but empty except for one person, the administrative manager. As soon as we walked in the door, she immediately stopped what she was doing and got up to greet us, directed us to some chairs, sat down with us, and started talking. "How are you? Don't worry; you are in the best hands. Everything will be all right. I think I know what you are going through, cancer has affected my family too." She was engaging, and before I knew it, she and Isabel were talking about my sister-in-law's cancer and her recovery, about Jessica's accident, and about the rest of our family. Isabel was also listening to her comforting words about the surgeon, his team, other patients' success, and the surgeon's bedside manner. The concern that had been etched on Isabel's face was beginning to fade. She was smiling and even laughing as the administrative manager put her at ease. This was so important to me. I realized that in order for me and my family to get through this challenge, Isabel had to be calm and in agreement with the choice of a surgeon.

While we were talking, the surgeon walked through the office. He stopped, introduced himself, and asked if we would mind waiting a few minutes because he had to make an unplanned call to a patient who lived overseas. He apologized and left the room. They say first impressions are lasting impressions, and in this case, that first impression told me all I needed to know about the surgeon and his team: They cared about me and my family. He was certainly self-assured when he approached us in the office, but imagine he actually *apologized* for keeping us waiting!

When Isabel and I sat down with the surgeon in his office, the first thing he did was review my test results and assure us that everything would be fine. We were now part of his family. He went through a presentation that I am sure he does with all of his patients, but his passion made it seem fresh and inspiring, and it was at this point that I really began to believe in him. His passion made me a believer for two reasons: First, I knew that I needed his skills and those of his team to help me beat my cancer. Second, people who know me generally describe me as passionate, and I like passionate people. When I speak to groups of young managers, my closing advice to them is "Do you want to make a career or a life for yourself? When you reach my age and look back on your life, do you want to know you have made a difference? If your answer is yes, then find what you are passionate about and pursue it with all of your energy. Dedicate your life to your passion!" I saw that passion in the surgeon.

The surgeon covered his own background; the anatomy as it related to my cancer; the benefits of robotic surgery; his specific surgical technique; his team (both surgical and support staff); and the reputation of the hospital where he practiced. He told me that he could perform my surgery on February 2, 2011. He then looked at Isabel. "Men will get anxious in this situation, and you have to keep him calm," he told her. He advised me that February 2 might seem far away, but that I should not be concerned. He assured me that the cancer would not spread while we waited for the surgery. The reason for the wait was that he wanted to give the prostate time to heal after the biopsy. He advised me *not* to be impatient and run out and get radiation therapy, because if my cancer came back after radiation he would not be able to help me. He said there was an appropriate time for radiation therapy, *after* the robotic prostatectomy, and only if my PSA levels became elevated again. (After radical prostatectomy or radiation therapy, rising levels of PSA indicate residual disease or recurrence.)[4]

As we got up to leave, Isabel started to speak to the surgeon. She spoke about how good she felt because of this visit and began to tell him about Dr. Sorosh Roshan, the physician who had delivered all three of our children—had been the first person to touch our three treasures. Isabel has always admired and trusted Dr. Roshan, and she told the surgeon that, like him, Dr. Roshan was Iranian. She felt comfortable that, also like Dr. Roshan, he would take care of her family. The surgeon smiled and asked Isabel if she knew what Roshan meant in Farsi. When she said "No," he explained that it meant "to the light." He looked at Isabel and said, "How appropriate that Dr. Roshan brought your children to the light of life!"

He gave me his personal e-mail address and cell phone number and then introduced us to one of the nurses on his team. She told me that the quickest way to gain control of my urinary function after the surgery was to begin doing Kegel exercises. Kegel exercises build up the muscles around the bladder opening. She explained how to do the exercise, saying, "I don't want you to crack nuts with your rectum; just tighten up easily, like you are holding back from passing gas." Her sense of humor and professionalism and the sense of family and support we were already feeling from the surgeon's team made me even more comfortable. Little did I know then how often I would contact this nurse for advice during my recovery, and she was always there for me. Later, during my recovery, Isabel and I often joked about not cracking nuts with my ass and it always made us laugh.

Walking back to the hotel, the air seemed cleaner, the sun seemed brighter, and our spirits were higher. Isabel said, "Everything is going to be okay; this surgeon will take care of you." I agreed that I thought everything would get better, but I also thought that *I* would ultimately be responsible for beating my cancer. I needed a plan, a surgeon I could believe in (which I had just found), and a lot of prayers and support, but my attitude and will would be necessary weapons if I were to succeed. The surgeon and his team would prepare me for the surgery, remove the cancer from my body, and support me in my recovery. Yet the question I still had to answer with my words and actions was, "Did I truly believe I would beat my cancer?"

My State of Grace

Believing in my surgeon and his team was not enough. I had to believe in myself and my ability to beat my cancer and get my life back. In the beginning there were many ups and downs; most of the time I did believe that I was going to beat my cancer, but occasionally, if only for a minute, doubt would creep in, and I would physically shudder at the thought of my cancer winning. One day right after our initial visit with my surgeon, however, I lost it and came dangerously close to a nervous breakdown.

I remember roaming aimlessly around the house, thinking, *Why not go out for a ride, get some fresh air and take your mind off of your cancer?* I went to the garage and took the car cover off of my pride and joy, my classic 1978 Porsche 911SC. I have loved Porsches since I was in college, and in 1996 I had been fortunate enough to purchase one. The appeal of the Porsche for me is its design and craftsmanship; the speed is nice, but design and craftsmanship have a higher priority. I like to take the Porsche out and drive around the neighboring towns just to relax as I shift gears and listen to the engine. My friends joke about seeing me with a smile on my face, driving my Porsche at fifty-five miles per hour as everyone passes me.

That day, as I drove through the neighboring town of Westfield, I decided to go to Fairview Cemetery to visit my father-in-law's grave. It wasn't uncommon for me to do this; Fairview is a beautiful, tranquil place, and my father-in-law had been a real treasure to me, so out of respect I would usually stop by for a visit. Close to his plot are the graves of three young adults who tragically died before they reached their twenty-first birthdays; one of the boys had been a friend of my oldest son, the girl had gone to school with my daughter, and the other young man had known my youngest son. My habit was to stop by my father-in-law's grave, tidy up the area, and then walk the grounds past the sites of these three kids. Again, this was my way of relaxing and, at the same time, getting focused on what was really important—enjoying life and family.

When I was done, I got back in the Porsche and drove home. I sat down at the table in the kitchen where Isabel was cooking. She turned from the stove and asked where I had gone, but I couldn't answer. All I could do was cry. She stood behind me, hugged me, and cried. We stayed that way for a long time. Attitudinally, that was my lowest point; I felt like everything was out of control. I had the best surgical team to believe in, yet everything seemed out of control.

A work-related event helped me regain the focus I needed. The week before Christmas, I took a vacation day to help Isabel with the last of our Christmas shopping. While shopping, I got a call from the office that there was an issue regarding an expense related to a holiday party planned at our California office. I listened to the details but then reacted in a not-so-pleasant way. A member of my staff later called back to apologize for having bothered me on my day off. He said the issue should not have come to my attention, and given "what I was going through," he was really sorry. He's a nice guy, and I knew he really did feel bad for "what I was going through," but his heartfelt and unnecessary apology made me think. What *was* I going through? Sure, I had prostate cancer, and the road ahead was going to be challenging, but did I believe I would survive and get my life back? If the answer was going to be yes, then I realized I had to live and think that way. I was determined to keep negative thoughts out of my mind. I would try to project calmness and return as best I could to my normal precancer life. I would not let my cancer change me!

Fast forward to the morning of February 2, the day of my surgery. The nurse who was taking my vitals noted my blood pressure; it was 107 over 70 (a very good number for someone just about to have major surgery). A few months later Jessica asked, "Dad, how did you stay so calm that morning? We were all nervous and you were so calm. When you left us to go upstairs to the operating room you smiled, kissed us, and told us you loved us, and then calmly walked away with mom."

On the day of my surgery, I was in a totally different state of mind than I had been in on the day I went for the ride in my Porsche. I like to say that I was now in "a state of grace!" What happened to me between that December afternoon and the day of my surgery? Certainly, believing more and more in my surgeon and his team helped me. The kindnesses, thoughts, and prayers of my friends and coworkers made a huge difference. On December 17, Nick had asked Jess to marry him and she had said yes, so the wedding was on. After three not-so-great events—Rem's cancer, Jessica's accident, and my cancer—our family's fortunes finally were heading in a different direction.

Yet something else had also happened to me. I had made a conscious effort to change the focus of my beliefs concerning my cancer and the future. Outwardly, I was saying all the right things, telling everyone that I was okay and that the surgery would be successful, but inwardly, I still had doubts creeping into my mind. After my near nervous breakdown in early December, however, I adjusted my attitude, and the rest of December and all of January were without incident. Other than the occasional visit with my physicians, my life was normal. I went to work every day and spent the evenings at home doing the same things I had done prior to being diagnosed. The one thing that did change was the joy that I felt every morning when I woke up. For as long as I can remember, upon waking up each morning I have thanked God for the day and prayed that I live up to my God-given potential. I have also prayed that I continue to be a person who cares about other people and their well-being. Now, the intensity of God's response to that prayer had changed, and I felt that I was now at the maximum of my potential, living a normal life, fighting my cancer, and caring about others. I was in my state of grace!

The Difference Between Trust and Belief

I want to explain the difference between trust and belief and why the distinction is so important. I think that when you are dealing with prostate cancer and the elite group of surgeons that treat this type of cancer, you can trust that anyone of them can handle your situation. After all, they are the best of the best, and they all have statistics to prove their capabilities. When I discussed these statistics with a friend, Mark, he stopped me and said, "Pat, the only statistic that is important right now is a sample size of one, and that one is you, so pick the surgeon who is right for you." I took Mark's advice seriously and determined that *right for me* meant the best of the best in terms of someone with the right surgical skills, someone who cared about me and also my family, someone who would be there whenever I needed them, someone to whom I could talk and ask questions (after all, there were going to be technical issues that I needed to understand), someone who understood my needs, and, above all, someone who was passionate about getting rid of my cancer. If you are fortunate enough to find that "someone," then you have to believe in them completely. You have to stop researching on the Internet and believe that the answers you are getting from your "someone" are the right answers for you. When family or friends give you advice on alternate therapies, you have to politely listen to them, because they love you and their intentions are good, but then you have to continue believing and following your "someone." Your job is big enough; you have to get your mind and body ready for the surgery and recovery. You do *not* have time for confusion or for second-guessing the path you've chosen. Let the "someone" you believe in help you with the rest!

Having said this, I can tell you that it is not that easy to believe in anything when you are dealing with cancer, but your beliefs grow stronger over time based on what you are experiencing. Isabel and I believed that my surgeon and his team were our "someone," and my surgeon and his team were getting ready to strengthen our belief in them!

I was driving home from work on December 16 when the story of Senator Ron Wyden (D-OR) came on the radio. The story described how the senator had recently been diagnosed with prostate cancer and would be missing key votes in the Senate because his procedure was scheduled for Monday, December 20. I am a political junkie, so the story would have held my interest if for no other reason than this was a lame-duck session of Congress and the votes on key bills were close, so every vote (including Wyden's) was important. Forget about politics, however; this was about prostate cancer. I remember cursing and screaming all the way home: why is *he* getting surgery so quickly and I have to wait until February?" When I walked in the door I told Isabel the story. I am sure I cursed everything from my cancer to my surgeon. When I finished, Isabel said, "Why not call the surgeon if you are concerned? But remember what he told us. He wanted to give the prostate time to heal after the biopsy. He said not to worry about the cancer spreading during this time. And he also told me, I was going to have to keep you calm because in these situations men get anxious." Isabel's logical approach and the power of my belief in my surgeon's advice prevailed; I calmed down and got ready for the holidays.

On January 2, I received a call from the surgical coordinator. She confirmed February 2 as the date of my surgery. I did not know it at the time, but she was about to become my "guardian angel." She made sure that everything I needed to do prior to being admitted to the hospital would be done, and done in an efficient manner. She was there whenever I needed her and answered all of my questions and concerns: "How do I get these test results to the surgeon?" "It looks like snow on February 2. Where can I stay that is close to the hospital?" No matter how many questions I had, she was always pleasant; she really understood what I was going through.

Another member of my surgeon's team called me on January 4 to review insurance coverage. I knew absolutely nothing about my insurance; Isabel usually took care of this in our family. The subject of insurance had come up only one time prior to this call; Holly and I had discussed it when we were researching which surgeon to choose. Holly had mentioned then that the surgeon we ultimately chose was not covered by our insurance plan, and I would personally have to pay more for the surgery. I had looked at Holly then with a straight face and told her, "I have already considered that. My out-of-pocket cost is less than the cost of all of the additional diapers I will need if I choose another surgeon!" The team member I spoke with now made all of the insurance information easy for me to understand, just as the surgeon had told me she would when he had spoken about the billing office team during our initial office visit. She and I talked about our families. Conversations like that, with real people, tended to put me at ease with my situation.

I mention these team members because they helped me in my time of extreme need. Their actions validated and increased my belief in my surgeon and his team. Several months later, I spoke with another patient of my surgeon who said, "You know, every time I call his office, I get a pleasant voice. I never get a voicemail or an automated directory. That is so important to me!" Obviously, my belief in my surgeon and his team was based on the fact that they were there for me and my family. The point I want to make here is that you have to find someone *you* believe in. Trusting that the surgeon can successfully perform the surgery is not enough. Believing and knowing that the surgeon and his team will be there for you and your family during the entire process, from presurgery to surgery to recovery, should be your goal!

ROBOTIC PROSTATECTOMY

Preoperation

On January 31, I left work around one in the afternoon. I tried to make my departure as normal as possible; I said goodbye and mentioned that I would see everyone in a few weeks. To be honest, however, with my surgery only two days away, I wasn't sure what the coming days would bring. I still had to buy a donut cushion to sit on after the surgery and the magnesium citrate (an over-the-counter bowel cleanser), as well as some diapers and pads. Isabel had volunteered to buy these items for me, but I felt I needed to buy them myself. After all, it was my cancer, and I needed to take ownership for everything, including my embarrassment over buying these items.

On the way to the medical supply store I called a friend, Dave, and joked about buying the donut, "explosives," and diapers. Dave's acceptance and participation in the humor helped me get through the afternoon. I realize now that I was entering my zone; I knew that I had done everything else I could do, and all that was left were these last-minute purchases, fasting the next day, and cleansing my bowels. I was determined to "walk the talk": to be calm and to lead by example with the hope that, as a result, everyone else would be calm.

When I arrived at the store to purchase the donut cushion, two women were there; one was an employee and the other a customer. I decided to stand by the register and wait my turn. The store employee interrupted her conversation with the customer and asked if she could help me, to which I responded, "Yes, but I'm in no hurry, so I can wait until you are finished with the other customer." She seemed a bit taken aback and asked again how she could help me. At that moment I realized that if I really was going to take ownership for my cancer and my situation, I had to speak up and do it now. "I need to purchase a donut cushion; the one you sit on after surgery. I am having prostate cancer surgery on Wednesday, and the surgeon recommended that I buy the donut cushion." For a moment, it seemed like all of the air was sucked out of my chest and the room.

I had done it! I had spoken up and taken ownership. My situation was real, and I took ownership! This might not seem like much to you, but it was big for me. I had planned everything in my mind. I had confronted every fear, and here I was, taking ownership and buying the silly donut from a woman while another woman listened in. There was no laughter, no jokes or smirks about this big guy buying a small round cushion to sit on. The reaction I did get was similar to what I would receive over and over again during my journey. The employee, in a kind and compassionate manner, told me, "I do not want to sell you that donut cushion; there is something so much better. You will be sore after your surgery, and given a man's anatomy, I recommend you go to a baby store and buy a Boppy*. It will do a much better job than the donut cushion."

When Isabel and I discuss encounters like this one, she is often shocked and finds it hard to understand my fears. She replies, "So what if the store clerk was a woman? You had to buy the donut cushion. What is there to be embarrassed about?" I think that my behavior is part of the bigger problem. Men are too proud. We think of ourselves as strong, and most are certainly private about certain

---

* A Boppy is a C-shaped pillow that offers an ergonomic way to nurse or bottle-feed a baby. When I went on the Boppy website, I got this wonderful feeling about the women and men of the company and their passion for improving the lives of mothers and their infant children. This feeling was reinforced when I saw my daughter utilizing a Boppy to care for our cherished granddaughter. I cannot help but think of the rule of unintended consequences: Who would have thought that the passion of the employees at Boppy would have impacted the life of a prostate cancer patient in such a positive and unique way?

issues. We have an irrational fear of intimacy. We need to step away from this type of behavior and get past our fear; this was one of my small steps. By the way, the store employee was right; I purchased a Boppy and found it very comfortable. The legend of the Boppy lives on; I have recommended it to many other men who agree with the store employee's assessment.

A snowstorm was forecast for February 2. We had planned for just such an event and had reservations at a hotel about ten blocks from the hospital. Plans like this were so important to my state of mind. If I had stayed at home and then had to travel into the city under those conditions, I am sure I would have been a nervous wreck. We arrived early on the afternoon of February 1 so that I could begin preparing for the surgery. The process was straightforward and easy to understand: no solid foods the day before the surgery, consume only a clear liquid diet, drink the bottle of magnesium citrate around three or four o'clock in the afternoon, and then have nothing to eat or drink after midnight. The room and the hotel in general seemed an out-of-place setting to me for these activities; I was cleansing my bowel for surgery in a boutique hotel that reminded me of weekend getaways to places such as San Francisco and Saratoga Springs. My lasting memory of the room is of the high ceilings in the bathroom and how the sounds associated with my cleansing resonated within them.

As it turned out, the weather forecast was correct. There was a major ice storm on the morning of February 2, which made the trip into the city very difficult for our son Damian, who was coming to be with us. My surgery was scheduled for noon, so at around nine-thirty Damian drove us to the preoperative unit of the hospital. I was born and raised in the New York metropolitan area and did my graduate studies in the city at New York University, so I was definitely familiar with New York City and New Yorkers. Yet even with this familiarity, I was not sure what to expect when I entered this prestigious "big city hospital." In the past I had visited this facility for business reasons, but now I was a patient. The guard at the entrance greeted us with a big smile and a "Good morning." He gave us directions to the preoperative service unit and told me he hoped everything worked out. Everywhere we went that morning, my family and I were treated in a professional, efficient, and caring manner. We were a little early, so we waited in a reception area. Jess and Sean arrived, and we sat around talking and laughing despite our nervousness. Dr. Luca, a cardiac surgeon who is a close friend, had driven in from New Jersey to be with us, and his being there had a calming effect. My family and I certainly appreciated that he had made the effort to get into the city to be with us.

Soon there were forms to complete, so time went by quickly. After completing the forms in the admissions area, Isabel and I were escorted to a private room where a nurse gave me the gowns I was to wear during the operation. She told me to put on the gowns and that she would return to check my vitals. When she checked my vital signs, she mentioned that my blood pressure was 107 over 70. While she checked my vitals, we spoke about our families and the weather. She really took the time to make us feel comfortable. That hospital may have been a "big city hospital," but for me it had a small town feel. The staff was wonderful! Everyone was so kind and pleasant. Our children joined Isabel and me when the nurse was finished. Our two sons were nervous, and even though they were thirty-four and twenty-four years old, they were into everything in the room. They argued about who was heavier and tried to get the electronic scale to work. Both Isabel and Jessica kept telling them to calm down and stop fooling with the scale, but to no avail. The three of us looked at the two brothers and just burst out laughing. Another nurse knocked on the door and told me that it was time to go upstairs for the operation. She said Isabel could join me, but only two of the children could go with us; only three family members were permitted upstairs. Damian offered to stay behind, but true to who my children are, they decided that they would all stick together and stay downstairs. I didn't know what the next hours would bring, but my children's affirmation of their love for each other was a great shot in the arm! I kissed each one of them, told them I loved them, and said I would see them later. Then Isabel and I went upstairs.

My surgeon met us in a room right outside of his operating room. It was comforting to see him, even more so because he was wearing his "game face." He can be pleasant and charming, but this morning he was all business. He checked my charts and told me he thought I had made a commitment to lose more weight. He had me lift my gown to see how big I was and then said something like, "You do not have a big gut. You are big everywhere. You will be fine." I wanted to say: "I'm not big, I'm pleasantly plump!" Instead I passed on the opportunity until the surgeon left and then told Isabel. Just as we started laughing, a member of the surgical team came into the room and told me it was time for the surgery. Isabel and I smiled and gave each other a kiss. "See you later!" I told her, and off I went to the operating room.

The Surgery

This is certainly one of the most important parts of my story, but the anesthesiologist put me under soon after entering the operating room, so my observations will be limited. If you asked people who work with me what I am like, chances are they would tell you that I can be direct and deliberate and that I love efficiency. When I entered the operating room, I was amazed because everyone seemed to have a purpose. There was no confusion or wasted effort. The team's actions were orchestrated, and their efficiency made me feel very comfortable. I lay on the operating table while they explained the various connections and monitors. The anesthesiologist identified the drug he would give me, Propofol, and said I may experience a warm feeling when he injected the drug. Another team member asked if I liked music. I remembered an article I had read about my surgeon; it mentioned he listened to music during surgery. The article mentioned Shakira, but the team member said today's choice was Christina Aguilera. It was a few minutes after noon when they asked me to begin counting backward from the number ten. I don't recall how far I got; my only recollection is a burst of warmth that started at my neck and quickly shot down through my circulatory system. In my mind's eye, it looked like the spacecraft Millennium Falcon bursting into action. Regardless, I was out.

Waking Up in *My* Heaven

I mentioned earlier that Isabel and I have a bungalow in Stone Harbor, New Jersey, where we go to relax and really enjoy ourselves. We purchased it in 2000, and it has proven to be not only a great place to which we can escape, but also a great investment. People occasionally ask me if I would sell the bungalow and realize the sizable appreciation in value. I always answer, "No. This is as close to heaven as I will ever get, and I have no plans on leaving heaven." So it was a pleasant surprise that when I woke up in the operating room to the anesthesiologist shaking me and calling my name, my first impression was that it was a sunny and warm day and that I was standing at the end of 110th Street in Stone Harbor, looking out on the Atlantic Ocean. I had woken up in *my* heaven!

Postoperation

My surgery took about an hour and a half. After an additional half an hour I was wheeled from the operating room to the recovery room. In the recovery room I felt surprisingly awake and aware of my surroundings. I did not feel any pain, and I was rapidly regaining my senses. The attending nurse realized immediately that I was feeling pretty good. As I struggled to sit up, I noticed an older woman in the bed next to me. I smiled and said, "Hi, how are you?" She smiled and answered, "Fine." The nurse noticed my movements. "You are a friendly one. Do you want to sit up?" she asked. I told her, "Yes, I am friendly and, sure, I would like to sit up." I suppose I was a bit curious; I had never been a patient in a recovery room. I did not know the outcome of my surgery, but I certainly was happy that it was over and that I felt so good. About fifteen minutes passed and then I saw two familiar faces: Dr. Luca and his friend Dr. Gabriele were at my bedside. (Dr. Gabriele who worked at the hospital is a personal friend of Dr. Luca; I had previously met him at medical congresses we both attended.) Dr. Luca has a contagious smile; it was so good to see them both. They commented on my color and how good I looked. Dr. Luca said, "If I did not know it, I could not have guessed that you just had surgery." We exchanged pleasantries, then they left the recovery room and went to let Isabel and my family know that I was fine. As I write this, I am reminded what a blessing Dr. Luca, Dr. Gabriele, and all of our friends are!

Two hours later Isabel joined me in the recovery room. By this time, I was wide awake and feeling great. We smiled and laughed when the nurse commented on my inquisitive nature. After a short time, my surgeon stopped by and said the surgery had gone as planned and was a success. That was all I needed to hear. I was elated, but Isabel was not. She asked if my cancer had spread. "Did you get all of the cancer?" He said we would have to wait for the pathology report, but Isabel was insistent. "Based on your experience, what do you think?" she pushed. "We have to wait for the pathology report," he insisted, but she would not let it go. Finally I told him, "Doctor, I have been married to Isabel for thirty-eight years, and I do not think she will give in. She wants an answer." He smiled. "I'll have an answer when the pathology report comes back. Now relax and get some rest. I will see you in the morning."

After about six hours in recovery I was moved to a private room. It was approximately eight o'clock in the evening. The kids had gone home, so we called to let them know everything was okay. My nurse was attentive to our needs. She got us something to eat, made sure we were comfortable, and suggested that maybe I would like to take a walk. The nurse, Isabel, and I walked the floor a few times, and then it was time for bed. I was feeling no pain, but I worried what would happen when the medicine from the surgery wore off, so I decided to take an over-the-counter pain killer. I knew that there were stronger pain medications available, but I was concerned both about the addictive nature of these drugs and one of their side effects—constipation. I knew that in two or three days I would be expected to have a bowel movement, so I stayed away from the stronger prescription medication. Fortunately I never really felt pain, and soon afterward I even stopped taking the over-the-counter medication.

As I look back on that day, I am amazed by my recovery time. I had had major cancer surgery performed under minimally invasive conditions by a skilled surgeon and his team with the help of a robot, and just six hours later I was already walking the halls of the hospital feeling stiff but pain free. It seemed as though I was dreaming even before I fell asleep.

I don't recall what I ate on the evening of my surgery, but the next morning I remember having solid food (scrambled eggs and toast). My new nurse made sure that I was comfortable and then got me up and walking. Between my walks I had visits from members of the surgical team. One of the team's nurses stopped by to see how I was doing and to explain the function of the drain that had been placed in my abdomen during surgery. It was there to remove fluids from the operative field, and the level of drainage would be monitored. When it reached an acceptably low level, the drain would be removed. I was concerned about the pain I would feel when the drain was removed, but she advised me simply to hold my breath during that procedure and it would be painless. She was, of course, correct. One of my major fears was scrotal/penile swelling or bruising, which I had read about and had heard about from a friend who had had robotic surgery a few years before me. His description of the swelling and bruising he experienced certainly had caused me to lose sleep prior to the surgery. However, afterward I was delighted that morning to discover that I was not experiencing swelling or bruising, nor did I experience either during my entire recovery.

A lot was happening the morning after my surgery, and as I look back, I find it interesting that I had *no* reason to focus on my five abdominal wounds. They were small openings, roughly patterned like a five on the faces of dice: two to the left of my bellybutton, two to the right, and one in the center directly below it. The wounds were painless and sealed with glue. The abdominal drain site was on the right side of my belly. I could not see it while lying down, but I knew it was there because I could see the tube and collection bottle when the nurse emptied it. I am thankful that there was no pain associated with that incision. I also had a urinary catheter, called a Foley catheter, which was held in place by a balloon in my bladder. A tube from it exited my penis and was attached to a small external collection bag. The catheter and the bag were painless but cumbersome; I was not used to moving around with this appendage hanging from my body, nor did I realize that I would be urinating so much. Catheters are a nightmare for most men, and many of those I speak to have questions about it: How does it feel? Will it pull out? What happens if the collection bag overflows? What happens if the tube catches on something while I am walking? I had these same questions myself, and over the next week, I would learn the answers to these and more I had not yet considered. For now, however, it was simply an unnatural appendage hanging from my body.

Soon, my nurse was preparing me to go home. She explained how to empty the collection bag, how to change the tape that held the catheter tubing in place, how to shower and wash my wounds, and which medications to take and when.* My surgeon stopped by to see how I was doing; he was pleased that I did not require prescription pain medication and that I was walking. He said that because I had passed gas and the abdominal drain had been removed, I would be discharged in the afternoon. Isabel continued her questioning regarding the surgery, and again, he insisted that everything had gone according to plan and that we had to wait for the pathology report. So around two o'clock in the afternoon, just twenty-four hours after my surgery was completed, I was getting into our car to go home. I was glad to be heading home but a bit nervous about being on my own. However, I felt that I was prepared to take care of myself thanks to the instructions Isabel and I had received from the nurses.

The ride from New York City to our home in Cranford, which is located in Central New Jersey, was uneventful. I was sitting comfortably on my Boppy as Isabel maneuvered the streets of Manhattan. The roads had been cleared of the previous day's ice and snow, and the sun was shining on us through the sun roof.

* I was sent home with a variety of medications: an antibiotic to avoid infection from having the catheter in place, a prescription pain medication, and another prescription drug in case I experienced bladder spasms as a result of my bladder being stretched (remember, my prostate, which had been below my bladder, was now gone). Fortunately, I did not feel a need for the prescription pain medication during my recovery. The first night at home I took some over-the-counter pain medication just in case, but it ultimately proved unnecessary. I also never used the medication for the bladder spasms; although I did experience some spasms, they were more interesting than painful. I took the antibiotic and did not get an infection from the catheter. In addition to these I was told to take an over-the-counter stool softener; my medical team had expressed concern that I should not force a bowel movement for fear of damaging the surgical area.

A WEEK WITH THE CATHETER

Learning to Live with the Catheter

About four months after my surgery, I met a man who had been recently treated for prostate cancer and had opted for a robotic prostatectomy. After his surgery, he had walked three miles a day during the week he had the Foley catheter in place. He was and still is my hero! My experience, although not bad, was nowhere near as good as that, but his experience certainly sets a high goal out for those who strive to overachieve.

Mentally, I broke my week with the catheter into three overlapping periods. The first period lasted a couple of days, which was the "learning to live with the catheter" period. The second I liked to call "having the first bowel movement after surgery," which, with any luck, would be a short period. The third period, "showering and cleaning the area of the incisions" would go right up to the last day. Thinking of the week in these separate periods allowed me to compartmentalize and break up the time. If I had specific goals that extended over that week, I would be more focused on the goals and the time would go by more quickly.

When I first got home, I thought of myself as an astronaut out for a spacewalk while tethered to life support on the mother ship. This analogy may seem a little over the top to some, given that an astronaut on a spacewalk floats in outer space, in a hostile environment, thousands of miles above the earth, whereas I was recuperating in the safety of my home connected to a urinary drainage catheter. Let me try to explain. Simply put, the catheter, as previously described, connects the bladder to a collection bag via a tube. That tube is held in place on the bladder side by an inflated balloon, and at the opposite end it exits the body and connects to a collection bag attached to the leg or hanging from a bedpost. Still not equal to a spacewalk, you say? Well, for most men here is the equalizer: The tube makes that connection by passing through the penis! I am willing to bet that ninety out of one hundred men who read that last sentence will shudder at the thought.* I agree that this reaction is irrational, and after experiencing the catheter for a week I would add that the fears associated with the catheter are mostly unfounded. This is one of those areas where communication with others who have experienced the catheter is so important, so many men myself included worry about the catheter when in actuality it is such a small part of the entire experience. My fears regarding the catheter were many. An incomplete list would include issues such as, if I catch it on the bedpost will it pull out? OUCH! What would it feel like? If my two golden retrievers jump up on me, and they pull it out? Again, OUCH!—maybe even an OUCH! OUCH! If both golden retrievers were involved! Does it hurt? How does it feel when it is taken out? And a real concern—how do I avoid infections?

In reality, living with the catheter was easy, just a little inconvenient. One inconvenience was that I had to sleep on my back to avoid tangling or pulling on the tube. Another inconvenience was

* I feel comfortable stating that "90 out of 100 men…would shudder" based on my conversations with many men who were recently diagnosed with prostate cancer. These men would call me to discuss my experience and inevitably in the conversation the subject of the drainage catheter would come up as well as many unfounded fears related to the catheter. One Sunday evening around 10:00 I received a call from one of these men. He was in a good frame of mind; he asked some technical questions and expressed a strong faith in his God, and I was impressed with his positive outlook. We spoke for about an hour. It was getting late, so I started to end the conversation by assuring him that I thought he had made sound decisions and that I was hopeful that all would be fine. He agreed. "Well, good night," I then told him, "and certainly call me if you have any questions or just want to talk." There was a short silence, and then he spoke. "Wait, what about the catheter?" he asked. I laughed and told him there was nothing to it, but I then asked him to tell me his concerns. We spent another half an hour covering his fears about insertion, removal, accidental pulling out, discomfort, and infection.

that I drank a lot of fluids and therefore drained a lot. (The catheter comes with two drainage bags; a small bag that secures to your leg so that you can move around and a larger bag that can be hung from your bedframe while you sleep.) If I had used the smaller drainage bag, I would have been emptying the bag every hour, so Isabel and I fabricated a way to hang the larger bag to the inside of a plastic wastepaper basket. This enabled me to move around the house while eliminating the need for me to empty the bag so frequently (See "Pee Caso"). As soon as I sat down I would cover the trash can with a towel so the only thing anyone would see was a small section of the tube exiting my pants through the hole we created in the side seam of the pant leg. One small step for man; one huge leap for Pat! Neither the bedpost nor the dogs ever pulled the catheter out, and I reduced the risk of infection by taking the antibiotic as prescribed and keeping the area where the tube exited my body clean. The catheter took a little time to get used to, but I had other more important goals that needed to be addressed.

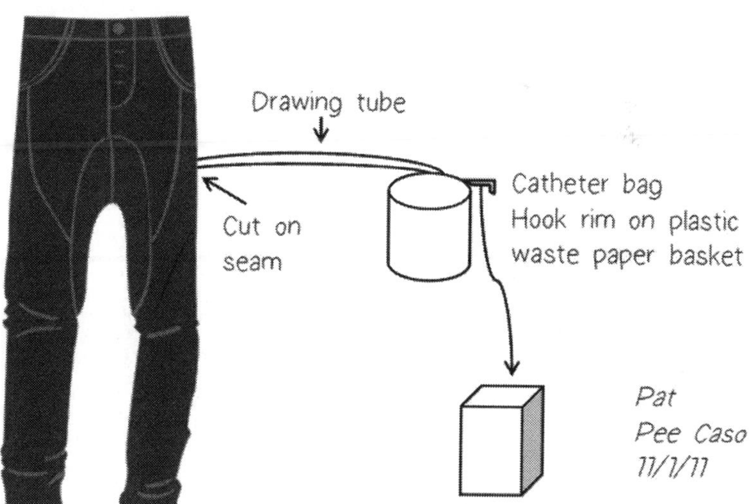

"Pee Caso." I sent this picture to a friend who had just had a robotic prostatectomy and was concerned about mobility while the catheter was in place. My friend is an artist and creative by nature, so I thought I would get into the act as well.

Having a Bowel Movement: Danger, Unexploded Bomb

One of the prerequisites to leaving the hospital was that I had to pass gas, not a difficult assignment given that I was bloated from the gas the surgical team had pumped into my abdomen during surgery. I think I passed gas as soon as I entered the recovery room! I was also draining urine freely with the help of the catheter. So the only task remaining for my bodily functions checklist was to have a bowel movement. When I left the hospital I was told that it was important that I have a bowel movement within three days of my surgery. I was also told that it was extremely important not to force the situation. The goal, as I understood it, was to have a bowel movement without exerting pressure on the surgical area. As I sat in the bathroom my thoughts drifted to a series I had watched many years ago on public television's *Masterpiece Theater* called *Danger UXB*.[5] The series had been about a British soldier, Lieutenant Brian Ash, whose job was to defuse unexploded bombs (UXBs) that had landed in Britain during World War II. The suspense grew as Lieutenant Ash was challenged to defuse the bombs each week without blowing up himself and the people around him. Like Lieutenant Ash, I remained focused on the task at hand, and on the second day, I finally was successful. I had a bowel movement without "blowing up" the area of the surgery. It was then that I realized that, for what I hoped would be a very brief period of my life, I was going to be a little too focused on "pee and poo." I was like a parent toilet-training his child, except I was the parent and the child. I would only be happy when I was fully "retrained."

Showering and Cleaning

The actual showering and cleaning were not that difficult. However, the physical act of showering and cleaning included overcoming the challenges of maneuvering oneself in a shower while wearing a drainage catheter and collection bag as well as carefully cleaning and drying the areas around the incisions (always pat, don't rub when drying). The initial shock of seeing the closed incisions on my body certainly set me back and reinforced the significance of what I had just been through. Part of my body had been removed because of cancer! On the positive side, however, I was in awe of the power of minimally invasive surgery. That was the first time I stood alone and realized the blessing that had been bestowed on me. My cancerous prostate had been removed through these little holes in my abdomen. Every time I showered during my recovery, I marveled at the miracle of minimally invasive robotic surgery and continued to dream of my successes that were still to come.

Untethered: The Catheter Is Out!

On February 9, Isabel drove me to my surgeon's office in New York to have the catheter removed. I was nervous about wearing the small drainage bag. Would it overflow? Would we get stuck in traffic? Most of all, I was nervous about having the catheter removed. Would it hurt? What happens if it gets stuck and will not come out? What happens if the balloon will not deflate? We were late getting to the office because of traffic, so Isabel left me at the door, and I went up to the office while she parked the car. I took the elevator upstairs and entered the office, and fortunately I was still dry. A nurse on my surgeon's team asked me to step into one of the rooms, drop my pants, and sit on the table. She was ready to remove the catheter. I sat there and closed my eyes; I was expecting the worst. After a few moments I asked when she was going to do it. "Mr. Walsh, it is out," she replied. I had not felt a thing! Now I was untethered and ready to move forward!

The nurse asked if I had brought a diaper with me. She instructed me to put the diaper on and explained the importance of doing my Kegel exercises to regain control of my urinary flow and get *out* of these diapers. This can all sound clinical and even comical, a man in a diaper (the potential opening for at least a few good jokes), but from my point of view this was my personal moment of truth: Could I accept the responsibility for my recovery?

RECOVERING

Responsible for the Future

With the drainage catheter out, it was clear to me that a shift in responsibility had occurred. Up to this point, most of the responsibility for the success of my surgery had been with my surgeon and his team. They'd had to guide me through the presurgery preparation and perform the actual surgery. I had been responsible only for my attitude and for following their instructions. Now, however, I was responsible for all of my future success. I had to continue to do my Kegel exercises, watch my weight, and most of all have a positive attitude. My surgeon and his team were there to answer questions and coach me, but the responsibility for a successful recovery lay clearly on my shoulders. (Although whatever was in front of me was my responsibility, in truth I was never alone. Isabel was always there to lend her support, to laugh, and to encourage me. Without her, I could not have succeeded!)

I was determined to get better and believed in my mind and heart that it was just a matter of time before I got my life back, which to me meant the following: First, I wanted to be a prostate cancer survivor. Second, I wanted my dignity—that is, control of my urinary function. Third, I wanted my manhood, meaning that after the surgery I wanted to be physically as close to the man I was before my cancer. This included the ability to have sex. If I came through the surgery as a cancer survivor with my dignity that would be great, but why not have bigger goals? I am a realist, so I knew that I was asking for a lot given the amount of cancer I had had (more on that later). I also realized that my recovery would not be a straight line from point A "the surgery" to point B "a normal life." I expected that there would be some setbacks along the way, so I was prepared for them if they occurred.

A Prostate Cancer Survivor

About four days after the surgery, my surgeon called me at home. The pathology report from my surgery indicated that I had had a lot of cancer. Cancer had been found throughout my prostate and seminal vesicles, which had also been removed. My lymph nodes, however, showed no sign of cancer. The surgeon informed me that I would require radiation treatment to ensure that he had removed all of the cancer. He explained that the radiation would be scheduled some time in May, after I regained control of my urinary function. (I was learning how strange this world of cancer could be: do your Kegel exercises, get control of your urinary function, and as a reward, you get radiation treatment!) He explained that there would be twenty-six low-dose treatments with no major side effects. I was disappointed, but I thought that this was a small price to pay to get rid of my cancer, so I moved forward.

Dignity: Control of My Urinary Function

This is where the drama takes place. Again, regaining urinary control is like toilet training a child, except you are both the parent *and* the child! There is only one way that I know of to achieve this goal, and that is to do your Kegel exercises regularly. I started doing Kegel exercises in early December 2010, and except for the period when I had the drainage catheter, I did them until mid 2012.* I tracked them in a notebook, following the adage that I followed in business:

* While the drainage catheter was in place, the surgeon's instructions were not to perform the Kegel exercises. I believe this was because of the potential damage the catheter could do to the stitches that rejoined the urethra. During surgery when the prostate is removed, the urethra is cut and then rejoined with sutures.

"What you measure is what you achieve." This is also a time when you will question your sanity. From very early childhood until I was diagnosed with my cancer, I never gave urine a second thought, except as a joke maybe. After surgery, however, controlling my urine became my obsession. I wanted to stop thinking about urine; to stop worrying about when, where, and how much I urinated; about where the men's rooms were; about what, when, and how much I could drink.

Like when you are a child, there are diapers and pads that you can wear until you gain control. It never bothered me to wear these diapers or a pad as long as I knew the situation was temporary. I have never met a man who likes to wear diapers or pads (or, as they are sometimes referred to, adjustable underwear or guards), but until you get control, you need them, and you thank God someone invented them. I made it a point to buy my diapers and pads myself. For me, it was embarrassing to stand in line with them in my shopping cart, but I used that embarrassment to motivate myself to stay focused on doing my Kegel exercises and gain control.

The first thing that struck me about urinating after the catheter was removed was the randomness of my urinary flow. (Like I said, being a prostate cancer survivor heightens your awareness of urine and its flow to a level you have probably never experienced before.) I think the stitches that rejoined the urethra during surgery as well as the weakness of the pelvic floor caused some of this randomness. Science aside, however, it can be laughable as well as frustrating. You aim for the center of the bowl and watch as you wash the wall next to the bowl. You feel a strong urge to urinate, then rush to bathroom and have only a mild drip. Worst of all, in my opinion: you finish urinating and zip up your pants, and then out shoots a gush of urine. That is when you hope you are wearing a diaper or pad. Frank, a close friend of mine, once mentioned that immediately after his robotic prostatectomy he realized that urinating became like driving a car, but not your own car! I have shared Frank's words of wisdom with many men; they all laugh and strongly agree. The good news is that as your body heals and you continue to do your Kegel exercises, you gain control, and life gets back to normal.

The coaching and support from my surgeon and his team were very important in helping me get control. All of the nurses on the team were just a phone call away, and their suggestions regarding what and how much to drink as well as when to stop drinking at night were instrumental. A great example of coaching was a conversation I had with one of the nurses about drinking alcohol. I had a bad habit that needed correcting, but until I spoke to the nurse, I didn't realize it *was* a bad habit. Prior to being diagnosed with my prostate cancer, I would have a glass of wine with my dinner. Being cooped up in the house after the surgery, however, I started having two glasses with my dinner. Then I started having a predinner drink about four days a week, usually a Manhattan, something unheard of before the surgery. When I spoke to the nurse about my sporadic, though improving, urinary control, she asked if I drank alcohol. She suggested that I stop drinking alcohol altogether for a month, because alcohol relaxes the muscles of your body. So I stopped for a month, and wouldn't you know it? My control increased dramatically. After the month was up I went back to moderate alcohol consumption, a glass of wine with dinner and a Manhattan on special occasions such as Thanksgiving or Christmas. This return to the consumption of alcohol has had no negative impact on my urinary control.

I began to regain control of my urinary function sometime over the summer of 2011. My control increased and my urge to urinate decreased over time, and as I write this I would say I am 99 percent in control. That 1 percent is still a challenge; when I lift heavy objects or make a quick movement I may have a drip. When I speak to other men who have had a robotic prostatectomy, these "accidents" seem to be common.

Manhood: The Ability to Have Sex

My concern regarding my ability to have sex was greatly reduced on the morning of February 27, 2011. I woke up to a familiar feeling: I had an erection. I was somewhat surprised because I had been taking the Viagra my surgeon prescribed on a regular basis but had forgotten to take it the previous evening. I was not able to see if all systems were working, because my surgeon's rule was "no sex for four weeks after the surgery."* I was excited and wanted to tell someone, so I sent my surgeon an e-mail: "I woke up this morning with an erection, assume this is good news!" When the four weeks passed, I immediately had sex, and everything worked fine, with one significant difference. I had an erection and the sensations of ejaculation and climax, but there was no semen. Imagine that, sex with no mess! The prostate and the seminal vesicles produce a significant percentage of a man's semen, so with nerves intact but no prostate or seminal vesicles, I was able to have sex without the cleanup afterward. I recognize that this lack of semen would not be the ideal situation for a younger man who wanted to have children, but for Isabel and me, it was just fine.

I was prescribed Viagra after the surgery. The first time I went to get the prescription filled was on February 14, Valentine's Day just by coincidence; given my surgeon's four-week rule this was strictly a clinical exercise and not an amorous adventure. When Isabel and I pulled to the drive-up window at our pharmacy, the young girl at the window looked at us and with a smirk on her face said, "Sorry,

* One of the first things you notice about my surgeon and his team is their professionalism. His professional appearance, the appearance of his staff, his office, even the literature he gives you is very professional. So I was surprised when I got the patient instructions regarding do's and don'ts after surgery. On the top of one of the typed pages was the handwritten instruction, "No sex for" what appears to be "*6 weeks* after your surgery." The number six was crossed out, and a four was written over it. As I look back, I wonder: was this a simple clerical error corrected with the strokes of a pen or did the wives, girlfriends, and significant others lose the vote to their husbands, boyfriends, and significant others?

we are all out of Viagra. You will have to come back tomorrow." I guess everything in life is a matter of timing! My understanding is that it is thought (although not clinically proven) that Viagra and other erectile dysfunction medication enhance the blood flow to the surgical area and help with healing. I stopped using the Viagra after about two months. It did not seem necessary for me because I could have an erection without it, although it did seem to improve urinary control. A few months later, I was asked by another prostate cancer survivor if I used erectile dysfunction medication. When I told him that I had used Viagra for a short period of time, he asked why I thought my surgeon had prescribed Viagra to me and Cialis to him. My response was that, given my age, he did not want me carrying two heavy bathtubs out to the backyard every time I wanted to have sex!*

The Day-to-Day Routine

With minimally invasive robotic prostatectomy, you can feel good soon after the surgery. In my case, after the urinary drainage catheter was out, I felt great physically, although I still needed to control my urinary function. I warn you, however: this feeling can be deceiving. You have to remind yourself that although only five small incisions are visible, your body has been through major surgery. You need to slow down and ease back into normalcy. I knew that given the weather and the time of year of my surgery, I was going to be in the house for an extended period of time. Prior to the surgery, I moved all of my tools out of the house. I did not want to be tempted to try some "small home repair" that could result in potential injury.

* The makers of Cialis currently run an advertisement on television that ends with a man and a women relaxing outdoors in two claw-footed bathtubs. I never fully understood the meaning, but maybe the wife thought she could tire her man out by having him carry two heavy bathtubs outside or possibly the man just wanted to show off his physical strength.

I also set up one of the empty bedrooms as a quiet space where I could relax, read, and have access to the Internet.

My recovery during the month after surgery went pretty much as planned. For the first few weeks I wore diapers; my urinary control was sporadic, so I thought the diapers were a better choice than pads. They were also a motivator; I did not like wearing them, and I knew if I wanted to get out of them I had to continue with my Kegel exercises and watch what I drank. My Kegel "routine" was as follows: I would start a Kegel, hold it for a ten count, relax for a five count, then repeat. I would repeat this nine more times. In a day I would do the "routine" ten times, so if you are counting, I did one hundred Kegel exercises a day (ten "routines" times ten equals one hundred Kegel exercises). I tracked my routines in a small notepad that I carried with me; my day was not complete until I did one hundred Kegel exercises. When I was out of the house and had to relieve myself, I would go into a stall in the men's room and after urinating I would do a routine. I took my recovery seriously, and my Kegel exercises were the foundation of my recovery. I found that as I gained control of my urinary function, everything else looked better. I also got into the habit of relieving myself every time I would get up from sleeping or sitting, even if I did not have a sensation to urinate. I also watched what I drank. I had one cup of coffee with a small glass of juice in the morning, approximately a liter and a half of water during the day, and tea in the afternoon. I controlled my intake of alcohol, and I did not drink anything after eight o'clock in the evening.

As my control improved, so did my courage. I started driving about a week after the drainage catheter was removed. I also went out to lunch with friends and family, remembering to relieve myself before I sat down and before I left the restaurant, even if I did not feel I had to go. I was getting anxious to return to work. I had made a point of not contacting my management team, because I was confident that they could run the business. In my absence, I had Frank, my vice president of operations, a trusted and capable friend who I knew could run the business, but still I wanted to get back to the job and the people I loved.

A Couple of Setbacks

Isabel and I went out for lunch on Thursday, March 4. We were celebrating my recovery and my planned return to work on the following Monday. I think it is important to comment on how well Isabel and I got along during my recovery. Some might think that we were celebrating the fact that I would be out of the house and out of each other's way. Nothing could be further from the truth. We actually enjoyed being around each other, and as my health improved, I tried to be less of a burden to her. I think I was successful. Isabel works from home and has an office in the house. We would see each other for breakfast, lunch, and, if she came downstairs, for tea, and then we would get together for dinner and a movie in the evening, laughing and enjoying each other's company. I treasured this time I got to spend with her. So, from my side, our lunch was truly a celebration of my recovery and Isabel's role in that recovery, my improved health, and my return to work.

The next day, Friday, I got up early and continued preparing for my return to work on Monday morning. As I cleaned up my desk and checked my clothes, I started to feel a chill, and then I started to shake uncontrollably. Around eleven in the morning, I told Isabel I did not feel well and went to lie down. I woke up around four in the afternoon feeling better, but not 100 percent. I thought I had flu. The next day, Saturday, I woke up again feeling better, but all at once, everything turned. The chills returned, and I had a 100-degree-plus fever. Isabel called my surgeon around four that afternoon, also thinking I had the flu and wondering if he could prescribe some medication. Instead, he instructed her to get me to a hospital.

We arrived at the emergency room around eight o'clock in the evening. By this time, in addition to my fever, I was having difficulty getting up from bed and—most distressing to me—losing control of my urinary flow. A CT scan of my pelvis was performed, and it was noted that I had an abscess that was pushing against my bladder. I was wearing a diaper, but I had forgotten to bring spares with me to the hospital—a big mistake. In the emergency room, I explained my situation to a nurse and asked him for a diaper to replace the one I was wearing. He returned with one that looked like a cloth for a small table. It was about two in the morning, and Isabel had gone home since I was going to be admitted, so I was on my own. I walked to the men's room and remembered how I had put diapers on our babies many years ago. Those early morning hours of March 6, 2011, were some of the lowest points in my journey. I was back in the hospital, having a difficult time getting out of bed, and losing control of my urinary function. The rest of the day was a blur to me. For part of the day I was on a restricted diet consisting of nothing to eat and ice to suck on. The hope was that a radiologist could insert a drain into the abscess. The procedure had to be rescheduled for Monday, however, so I was switched to a liquid diet.

My urologists stopped by to see me on Monday morning. They explained the procedure that the radiologist was going to perform and assured me that I should regain urinary control after the abscess was drained. The role of my urologists as well as all of my attending nurses cannot be overstated. Remember, up until my surgery, I had never been in the hospital. Now, there I laid, unable to get up on my own, barely a month after prostate cancer surgery, dependent on the competencies and kindness of so many. This was very strange to me. All of my life I had prided myself on my ability to get through any situation with my will and desire, but as much as I wanted to get up and get better, I could not do it alone. I feel it is important to say this, because these doctors, nurses, and support staff are special people. They see human suffering every day and continue to reach out and help people in need. This is personal. Thank you!

The insertion of the drain on Monday was an interesting procedure. Another CT Scan was performed to locate the exact position of the abscess, and then a needle and drain were inserted into it. I can make this sound pretty straightforward, but it wasn't that easy for me. First, I could not get off the gurney on my own, so a wonderful nurse helped me get up and onto the CT table. I was embarrassed by my lack of urinary control, but she assured me not to worry; after all, this was a hospital. It turned out that she lived in Kenilworth, the town where I grew up. We shared our memories for a bit, and then the radiologist mentioned the needle. The nurse must have seen the helpless look on my face, so she instinctively took my hand and assured me everything would be fine. One of my urologists had joined the radiologist, and when the needle perforated the abscess I heard a collective, "Ugh! That doesn't look good!" Over the next days the abscess drained continually. I was sent home on Wednesday with the drain, and for the next week I emptied the drain myself until a nurse from my surgeon's team removed it on March 18. The good news was that as the size of the abscess decreased, I regained more and more of my urinary control. By the time the drain was taken out, I was ready to resume my life and get back to work three days later, on Monday, March 21.

When I went to bed on the evening of March 18, I felt like a hot dog on the grill at a 7-Eleven. I rolled around all night, and around two o'clock in the morning, I got up and went to sleep in another room. After all, Isabel had been under a lot of stress, and there was no reason for her not to sleep just because I couldn't. No matter what position I was in, I just could not get comfortable. In the back of my mind, I knew what was happening: my kidney stone was moving. I tried to ignore it and hoped it would go away. By the evening of March 19, however, I was back in the emergency room, and just as I'd suspected, it was a kidney stone. I had passed a stone once before about three years earlier, and it had been the most painful experience I had ever had. After everything I had been through now I thought, *Lord, why are you doing this to me?* So much for never questioning. As it turned out, the stone was smooth in structure, and fortunately it passed relatively painlessly the next morning.

A RETURN TO NORMALCY

Back to Work

On Tuesday, March 22, forty-seven days after my surgery, I returned to work. My urinary control was not perfect, so I wore protection. My fears were many. I was concerned about the commute: a forty-minute ride on heavily traveled roads. What would happen if I got stuck in traffic? Could I control myself until I got to work? At work, what would I do if I was standing in front of people and suddenly sprung a leak? Luckily, none of my fears were realized. Yes, I got stuck in traffic, but I was able to control myself until I reached the men's room. I never leaked in front of people, although I will admit this was a fear I had for a long time. Isabel commented that she noticed that from time to time I would look down at my pants to check for leaks—old habits die hard. Being back at work was the perfect distraction. As I became more and more immersed in my day-to-day responsibilities, I spent less time thinking about my urinary control, and that control greatly improved. One of my goals was to return to work and not miss a beat. I wanted to get back to running a business. I was, after all, the president and chief executive officer of a large business with many responsibilities. Another one of my goals was to lead by example. I knew that many people were aware that I was now a cancer survivor, and I wanted to show them that I was still able to live a productive and happy life. Other than leaving work early the first few weeks, I resumed my normal routine. If you did not know about my cancer, I do not think you would have learned about it from my behavior.

The Underwear Bomber and Me

One of the first things that I wanted to do was to visit my team in San Jose, California. My business was divided into two groups, with approximately half the team in Wayne, New Jersey, and half in San Jose. My permanent office was in Wayne, but I liked to visit San Jose every six weeks, something I had not been able to do for approximately five months as a result of my postdiagnosis travel schedule and my cancer treatment. My main concern with the trip was to make sure that my team in San Jose was operating efficiently, driving innovation, and implementing our strategies. In addition to these professional concerns, I was faced with some very real personal concerns. The first was getting through airport security with my diapers and pads, and the second was maintaining control during a five- to six-hour flight. I am an optimist by nature, but the thought of being singled out at security as the next "underwear bomber"* or of losing control while trapped in my seat on a plane played some wicked games with my mind. Although I was wearing a pad and carrying spares in my bag, I got through security without issue. I always flew business class with an aisle seat, so the fear of having to disturb another passenger every time I wanted to get up went away, but I was still concerned about what would happen if the "fasten seat belt" sign went on and I had to go. I managed fluid intake and made a trip to the toilet every hour, just in case. I was self-conscious about getting up that much, but it was better to be safe than sorry! I had this

* When I traveled, I made sure I had enough diapers and pads for the entire trip, but at the same time, I prayed my diapers and pads were not exposed as I passed through airport security. I always worried that I would be stopped and questioned about what these diapers and pads were and why there were so many in my luggage. I especially worried about international travel. It would be difficult enough to explain in my native tongue, but imagine trying to do that in another language! When full-body scans were initiated at airports (partially as a result of the "underwear bomber" who had had explosives in his underwear), I really became anxious every time I went through airport security. Imagine: "Sir, please step out of line. What is it that you have in your underwear?" This was all the more reason to resolve my control issue as soon as possible.

running joke in my head that another passenger would notice that I was getting up so much and observe that maybe I had prostate problems and that I should have it checked. My reply would be a simple, "Been there, done that."

This trip to San Jose (and I am happy to say all of my plane trips since the surgery) was without incident; none of the feared events happened. As I gained more and more control, I made many West Coast and transatlantic trips with fewer and fewer visits to the toilet. Before leaving this topic, I want to mention two important lessons I learned. First, these fears can play games with your head. I had major business issues to deal with—sales growth, innovation, gross margins, and employee morale, to name just a few—while at the same time, the fears of leakage and becoming the next "underwear bomber" were real possibilities to me. I managed to do my job and deal with these fears by having a positive attitude. I recognized that I was getting better every day and that the control issue, the diapers, and the pads were temporary. I realized that getting better was my responsibility. This knowledge motivated me to do my Kegel exercises and get control of my urinary function. The second lesson I learned is related to urinary control the day after you fly.

When I arrived at my hotel in Santa Clara on my first West Coast trip, I noticed that my urinary control had diminished. The next day was more of the same, and to say the least, I was frustrated. By the second day after the flight I was back to my normal level of control, but the day after my flight home I had again the same pattern of diminished control followed by a return to normal. I probably would not have thought much of this pattern, but then I got a call from Pat, a nurse at my insurance company. Pat called from time to time to see how I was doing and provided advice and coaching. I have heard a lot about the impersonal nature of insurance companies, but the idea of having people like Pat available to help is a great idea. She was so supportive and contributed to my success. After my return Pat called and asked how my first trip to San Jose had gone. Then she asked a very specific question: "How was your control the day after the flight?" I was amazed and asked her how she knew that my control had changed. She explained that when you are in a pressurized plane for a long flight, your body retains water. (Have you ever noticed how difficult it is to put your shoes back on after a long flight because your feet have swelled?) The day after the flight, your body releases that water; hence my lack of control the next day as my body released what it had retained during the flight. Recently I spoke to another prostate cancer survivor who had just arrived in Disney World for a vacation with his family. He told me that he was frustrated because he had lost control and what had been planned as a celebration was turning into an ordeal. I mentioned the lesson Pat had shared with me, and his spirits picked up. The rest of the vacation was, I am sure, a success.

A Dream Realized

During my recovery, I believe it was in February, I had a terrible day. I cannot remember anything specific, but it probably had to do with some combination of the following: my aim in the bathroom, dripping, diapers, pads, or just plain old cabin fever. It was one of those days where you just want to scream, "I want my life back!" That night I had a dream that I was at the beach in a bathing suit with no diapers or pads and that I was getting ready to go swimming. I do not pretend to be an interpreter of dreams, but I think my dream was saying the obvious: I just wanted to be normal. Fast forward to August of the same year. I was at the beach in Stone Harbor with Isabel, Damian, and Damian's girlfriend. Damian asked if I wanted to go into the ocean for a swim. He has loved the ocean ever since he was a child; we had always had to fight with him at the end of the day to get out of the water. I am just the opposite. I will usually stand on the shore, content to get my feet wet, but on this day I agreed, and we both ran into the ocean. When I got out of the water, the dream from February immediately came to mind. I was overcome with joy. I told everyone that I was going back to the house for a minute. When I got back to the house, I sent my surgeon an e-mail titled, "A Dream Realized." In it I told him about the dream and thanked him for all of his help during the surgery and my recovery. Believe me, I wish no one would ever get cancer, but everyone should experience the feeling I had that day at the beach!

The Day I Got My Life Back

If you have been following my progress as documented in this book, I cannot blame you if you think I am somewhat crazy. It is not normal for a man to spend so much time focused on urinary control, diapers, and pads. You would be right. No normal man should spend time thinking about such things, but my prostate cancer temporarily took my normalcy away. Until I got it back, I had to focus on these things. So it is with much joy that I now arrive at Sunday, September 11, 2011, the Sunday after Labor Day. I was home in Cranford, sitting on the sofa watching the Sunday talk shows and reading *The New York Times*, when a thought occurred to me. I was not wearing a diaper or pad, I was enjoying a cup of coffee, and in the back of my mind, there were no thoughts about urine—none whatsoever. I went downstairs and gave Isabel a big hug and thought to myself, "Finally, I have my life back!"

The Big Day: Jess and Nick's Wedding

It is hard to describe how I felt about Jessica and Nick's wedding; joy and happiness are certainly a good place to start, but this wedding was so much more. Our family had been through so much in the year leading up to the wedding: my sister-in-law Rem's colon cancer, Jessica's bicycle accident, and my prostate cancer. Once Jess accepted Nick's proposal, however, our collective focus shifted to the wedding. Sure, my cancer was on my mind, just as I am sure Rem's was on her mind, but as a family, we were primarily focused on happiness: Nick and Jess's wedding. I am sure that planning for the shower, buying Jess's gown, and all the other special things that needed to get done kept Isabel going and certainly made her happy. My goal had also changed. No longer was I just focused on being there to walk my precious daughter down the aisle; that was a given. I was now focused on all of the days after the wedding when our expanded family would celebrate holidays, birthdays, and possibly the birth of grandchildren.

When the day, October 8, 2011, came, everything was flawless. Planning a beach wedding for the beginning of October is a gamble, but the weather was perfect and the ceremony went off without a hitch. Around four in the afternoon, Jess and I left the hotel and walked across the street to the beach, where the ceremony would take place. When I gave Jess to Nick and sat down next to Isabel, I was so happy to be alive and so proud of my family.

OPTIMISM: THE MEANING OF IT ALL

No Wax Prostate, Not Even a Wax Walnut or Doughnut

My initial reaction to my cancer was fear—fear for my life, fear that if I survived my cancer everything else in my life would change, and fear of all of the things I didn't know. When faced with other challenges in my life, I had addressed them with a mixture of four core beliefs: My belief that everything will always work out. My belief in a God that does not make mistakes. My belief in the power of prayer. And my belief in the power of a good sense of humor. When I was diagnosed with my prostate cancer, however, I was dazed and, for a while, ignored these beliefs. My first step toward recovery was returning to those beliefs. During the weeks after my diagnosis, I found myself thinking negatively about my cancer, daydreaming about how it would impact my life and my family. For example, I would think of the surgery and imagine my surgeon telling me the cancer had spread, that there was nothing more to do, and that I should go home and get my affairs in order. I would see the faces of Isabel and the kids and just freeze in place. These daydreams were unproductive and, as I learned, unfounded, but their impact was very real. I would become depressed and to an extent paralyzed, not wanting to move or do anything.

One day in December, around the time I took responsibility for my cancer, I remembered a prayer: "Lord Jesus Christ, make haste to help me do your will in my life, rescue me, and save me." From that point on, every time this negative daydreaming started, I would silently recite the prayer, and the negative thoughts stopped. Actually there were times when I found myself saying the prayer and realizing that a negative thought was coming on, although not yet actually there. Prayers such as this are powerful influences in my life, and in this situation, they proved to be just what I needed to help me get past the paralysis of negativity and fear and get on with the optimism that my treatment and recovery would be successful. I built on this prayer and my belief in a God that does not make mistakes. I started to believe that if God was presenting me with this challenge of my cancer, it was for a reason, and everything would be okay. I became more relaxed and focused on my responsibility and the future. My belief in a God that does not make mistakes and the power of prayer are very personal. I was raised a Roman Catholic, but I do not attend church or strictly adhere to the teachings of the church. This is sometimes described as a nonpracticing Catholic. This description sounds too negative to me. In a simple way, I do practice my faith and what the good Sisters of Saint Dominic taught me. I ask myself if my intentions are unselfish, and then I follow the Golden Rule—I treat people as I would like to be treated. I hope people who know me would say that I am trustworthy, that I tell the truth, and that I treat people respectfully, kindly, and lovingly. The reason I mention the private nature of my faith is because I was not prepared for, nor did I realize, the amount and power of the prayers of others who so thoughtfully cared about me and my family. They truly comforted us in our time of need.

In the fall of 2011, I was in Lisbon, Portugal, on business at a medical conference. I was traveling with a coworker and close friend, Jim. We had the weekend off, so Jim and I decided to visit Fatima. Fatima, Portugal, is a sacred site for Catholics where the Blessed Virgin Mary appeared to three shepherd children in 1917. Pilgrims visit this site to ask for blessings related to their problems. Jim is a wonderful travel companion; he is as knowledgeable as any professional tour guide, and his spiritual nature was a perfect fit for our destination. When we arrived at Fatima, we were impressed with the church and shrine in the center of town, but I personally thought the commercialism was a little over the top. There were shops that sold everything from religious medals and holy cards to baseball caps with the Blessed Virgin Mary on the front. The shops also sold wax body parts that the pilgrims offer with their prayers to the Blessed Virgin Mary. When I entered a store I noticed wax breasts, colons, legs, arms, intestines, and brains, but no prostate. Not even a wax walnut or doughnut that could be used as a proxy. I thought to myself, "What about me?" In lieu of a wax prostate, I bought half a dozen foot-long candles to offer at the shrine for the intentions of close friends as well as for men like me who were battling prostate cancer. As Jim and I drew closer to the shrine, the heat from its offering fire was intense. I saw a woman with a six-foot candle that was leaning in the heat. I looked at Jim and said, "And I thought I had problems." Jim just shook his head.

After we said our prayers and made our offerings, Jim checked with a guide and found out that the actual sites of the Blessed Virgin's visits were a few miles outside the center of town, so we decided to walk over and make a visit. The walk was relaxing, just two friends talking about human nature, spirituality, family, and the beauty of the surroundings. When we reached the site of the initial appearance, we commented on the calm that permeated the site. For a time we just sat quietly taking in the atmosphere. As we walked back to town, I contemplated the power of God, the beauty of life, and how lucky I was to be alive and to have so many friends like Jim.

A short time after my return from Fatima, Isabel and I had dinner with our close friends Kathy and Dave. Dave and I had worked together some twenty years ago, but we remained close friends, and we speak about once a week to catch up and joke about the absurdities of life. Dave knows my sense of humor better than anyone, and when I kid about my prostate cancer or my recovery, he always cautions me, saying, "You haven't learned yet? You are still crossing the line of acceptability. I can just see the Lord looking down on you and saying, 'When will this guy learn?'" Kathy shares David's sense of humor, but she comes from a close and devotedly Irish Catholic family.

Over dinner we talked about my recovery as well as my trip to Fatima. I mentioned the wax offerings and the lady with the six-foot candle. Kathy listened, laughed, and then mentioned that she had been saying a novena for me to Saint Peregrine, the patron saint of cancer patients, ever since I had been diagnosed. She also gave me a Saint Peregrine medal, which I wear as a reminder of the healing power of God, the warmth of true friendship, and the grace both have given me. This wasn't the first time that my humor and faith seemed to be in conflict, so I said to Kathy, "You know I appreciate and am thankful for your prayers. And I mean no disrespect because I share your beliefs. But for me, sometimes I have to laugh at my situation, my cancer, and my faith in order to get by." I also mentioned that I believed God gave me my sense of humor so that I could get through difficult situations such as these. Kathy smiled and shook her head, very much as Jim had done at Fatima, maybe to agree, or more likely to say, "I will keep praying for you. You need it."

Please understand that the specifics of my beliefs are not what is important here. What is important is that at times in my journey, I needed some spiritual support as well as the support of my friends. I believe it would have been impossible to successfully make the journey without this support.

Still Traveling

As I look back on the time since that day in December 2010, when I first took responsibility for my cancer, I can honestly say that every day has been better than the day before. Sure, there have been some setbacks both major and minor, as well as moments when I would scream out that "I want my life back." In the end, however, I got my life back and it is even better than it was before. I also recognize that my journey with prostate cancer is not over. I live with the knowledge that if any of my blood tests come back with a PSA level other than nondetectable there will be a concern that my cancer is still with me. If that were to happen I would require radiation therapy and potentially other treatments. I like to believe that if my cancer returns, modern medicine and optimism will overtake fear and everything will be okay.

Realizing Life While We Live It

It may be hard for some to believe that my life after cancer is better than it was before, but it is true. The best way I can describe it is to quote from the play *Our Town* by Thornton Wilder. In the play, a girl Emily dies at a young age, and after dying she is allowed to leave her grave and return to her parents' house in Grover's Corner to observe the life she loved so much. While she is observing, she has the following conversation with the Stage Manager, another character in the play.

> *Emily to the Stage Manager:* "I didn't *realize*. So *all* that was going on and we never noticed! Take me back—up the hill—to my grave. But first: Wait! One more look! Goodbye! Goodbye, world! Goodbye, Grover's Corners—Mama and Papa—Goodbye to clocks ticking—and my butternut tree! and Mama's sunflowers—and food and coffee—and new-ironed dresses and hot baths—and sleeping and waking up!—Oh, earth, you're too wonderful for anyone to realize you."
>
> *She looks toward the stage manager and asks abruptly, through her tears:* "Do any human beings ever realize life while they live it?—Every, every minute?"
>
> *Stage Manager:* "No—" *he pauses.* "Saints and poets maybe—they do some."

Before you get the idea that I am getting too full of myself, please recognize that I do not consider myself a poet or a saint—in fact, I'm far from those things. I am just a regular guy who, among other things, now shuts off his iPhone and iPad during conversations. I consciously try to listen to others, enjoy their company, and realize more often than not that the most important time is now, the most important people are the ones we are with, and the most important thing is LOVE.

The Jewel of Optimism

Many times, I have questioned the other changes in my life. Why contact recently diagnosed men and spend hours discussing my experiences and their concerns regarding prostate cancer? What qualifies me to write a book about prostate cancer? Am I doing these things for selfish reasons, just because it makes me feel good? Initially, I based my decision to reach out to others on the belief that who better to talk about prostate cancer than me, a survivor? I was broken, and now I am fixed. One night over dinner I discussed this with a friend, Dr. Daryoosh, a skilled cardiac surgeon with a wonderfully thoughtful and poetic nature. When I explained my thoughts to Dr. Daryoosh, he said he understood but that maybe I should consider looking at things more positively. Yes, I had had cancer, but humans do get cancer, so I was not broken; I was just a human with cancer. He suggested that I had been given a gift, "a jewel." He asked me to consider what that jewel was. I thought for a while and then answered, "This jewel was me surviving my prostate cancer with my optimism intact." We agreed that my recovery and my optimism are the gifts, the jewels that I should share with others.

A simple phone conversation cleared any remaining doubt I had regarding reaching out to men and writing this book. In the fall of 2011, on Halloween to be exact, I was told that I was being terminated from my job (this gave me a whole new understanding of trick or treat). The termination was the result of business consolidations, reorganizations, and acquisitions, all professional situations, which up until now I was in charge of managing, but now I was the one out of work. As with my cancer diagnosis, I was not inclined to ask "Why me?" when the termination happened. I had never sought a reason for the good things in my life, so again I was not going to ask the reason for the bad. I accepted the fact and began to prepare for the future and what would be next in my life.

My employer told me that if I had any questions regarding my benefits I should contact Janice from the human resources department. One day in March 2012 I called Janice to ask a question regarding my insurance coverage. Being the wonderfully caring person she is, Janice asked me how I was doing, and I told her that in addition to looking for a job, I was reaching out to men recently diagnosed with prostate cancer while writing a book about my own experiences. I told her that I wanted to raise awareness and hoped to change men's behaviors regarding prostate cancer. I knew that there had been more layoffs at work, and I recognized how stressful Janice's job must be, so I apologized for the life I was leading. I was concerned that her perception might be that I was collecting severance while selfishly sitting at home and writing a book about my personal experience, and meanwhile she and her team were busy tending to the needs of the really needy—the laid-off employees and their families. Janice did not say much while I apologetically described my situation, but immediately after our call ended she sent me the following message in an e-mail: "Thank you for sharing with me what you are doing with the support for other prostate cancer patients. My grandfather passed away from prostate cancer many years ago. He never went to the doctor, even though he had very bad symptoms, and by the time he was finally diagnosed, it was too late. What you are doing is a wonderful thing." My reaction to that e-mail was that my actions are *wonderful,* possibly, but *necessary,* certainly!

EPILOGUE

As I complete the writing of my book, I have had approximately twelve blood tests for the presence of PSA. Each test has returned as "PSA level nondetectable" (mandatory "knock on wood"). On the one-year anniversary of my surgery, my surgeon cautioned me that given how much cancer I had had, the PSA could rise, and if it did I would then need the radiation treatments. Right now, I have no signs of PSA, and therefore I have not had the radiation treatments. After radical prostatectomy or radiation therapy, rising levels of PSA indicate residual disease or recurrence.[6]

I feel the need to explain why I wrote that I have had "approximately twelve blood tests." The reason is that I do not know how many blood tests I have had since my surgery. I don't focus on the number of tests—that's the past. With my cancer, I try to focus only on today. The only time I focus on the blood test is during the period between the test and when I get the result. Isabel has commented that I act differently and get anxious while waiting for the result.

After my surgery, I met a man at my surgeon's office. He was recently diagnosed with prostate cancer and was in the process of determining how to treat it. He asked me, "After your surgery, do you feel you are cured?" to which I answered, "No. I consider myself a prostate cancer survivor; if I were cured I would not have to have routine blood tests to check for the presence of PSA." He then asked, "Then why bother with the surgery if you are not cured?" My reply was simple. I live my life to the fullest, recognizing that today could be as good as life gets so why waste the day worrying about whether I am cured or a survivor?

Pat Walsh

Winter 2014

APPENDIX ONE
TIMELINE OF EVENTS

Date	Event
6/30/2000	The first time I heard about prostate-specific antigen (PSA) was in a note from my internist after a routine physical. There was a simple note under the tests that were normal, "P-S-A," and no level was given. I was fifty-one years old.
6/26/2002	After the next routine physical examination, my internist's notes show a normal PSA level of 3.3.
9/28/2004	After yet another routine physical examination, my internist's notes show a PSA level of 4.6 with a reference to less than 4.5 being normal and a recommendation that I see a urologist.
12/04/2004	I see a urologist for the first time; I have a PSA test and a digital rectal exam (DRE). My PSA level is 3.3, and the DRE results are normal. The urologist recommends a biopsy, but I refuse and decide to monitor my situation.
2005–2009	I have eight PSA and DRE examinations with this urologist during this time, and my PSA level ranges from a low of 3.1 to a high of 7.3 (I never followed up with him on the last test, but I believe it was 7.3). All of my DREs are normal. After each exam the urologist recommends that I have

a biopsy, and each time I refuse and continue to monitor my situation.

Mid-2009 After the last routine PSA blood test, my urologist leaves me an urgent phone message to contact him because my level has spiked. *I never return the call.*

9/2010 I have an appointment with a new urologist. My DRE is normal, and I schedule a PSA blood test for the following week.

10/2010 The results of my PSA test are 7.3. My new urologist also recommends a biopsy. I refuse and express the desire to keep monitoring my situation. The urologist listens and then tells me, *"Mr. Walsh, you have cancer, and you will not let me prove it to you."* I agree to have a biopsy.

11/19/2010 I have my first and only biopsy.

11/23/2010 "Mr. Walsh I am sorry to tell you but you have prostate cancer."

11/25/2010 On Thanksgiving Day, only my wife Isabel and I know that I have cancer. We decide to let the family know after the holiday. My daughter's boyfriend tells me he will ask my daughter to marry him.

11/28/2010 I tell the children that I have been diagnosed with cancer, one of the hardest days of my life.

12/2010 Isabel and I meet with my urologist to review the results of the biopsy. Cancer is present in eight of the twelve biopsy cores. My urologist recommends that I have robotic surgery to remove my prostate.

	He gives us a list of potential surgeons and schedules computed tomography (CT) scans and a bone scan for me to see if the cancer has spread.
12/3/2010	I receive the good news that the scans are negative the cancer has *not* spread.
12/8/2010	We first meet with my surgeon. The surgery is scheduled for February 2, 2011.
1/31/2011	This is my last day at work before my surgery.
2/2/2011	I have surgery, a robotic prostatectomy.
2/3/2011	I leave the hospital just twenty-four hours after the completion of my surgery with a urinary drainage catheter in place.
2/10/2011	I return to the doctor's office to have the urinary drainage catheter removed.
2/14/2011	On Valentine's Day my surgeon gives me a prescription for Viagra, an erectile dysfunction medication, with the hope that the medication will increase blood flow to the area of the surgery and promote healing. When Isabel and I go to pick up the prescription at the pharmacy, we are told, "Sorry we are all out of Viagra, please come back tomorrow." Timing is everything!
2/27/2011	I forget to take the Viagra but wake up with an erection. However we do not have sex until early March because of my surgeon's "four-week rule": no sex until four weeks after the surgery.
3/5/2011	I go to the emergency room of the hospital with a fever. I am admitted with an abscess that is pushing against my bladder.

3/7/2011 — A drain is inserted into the abscess, and I am released from the hospital and sent home with the drain exiting from my side. The abscess continues to drain for another week.

3/18/2011 — The drain is removed.

3/19/2011 — I am admitted to the hospital for a kidney stone, which I pass the following morning.

3/22/2011 — I return to work after forty-seven days of recovery.

9/04/2011 — I have a wonderful revelation: I have my life back!

10/8/2011 — Jess and Nick are married on a beautiful, sunny, and joyous day at the beach. We celebrate our happiness with family and friends!

APPENDIX TWO FREQUENTLY ASKED QUESTIONS

Once again I feel the need to state my personal disclaimer. I am a person, and I was a prostate cancer patient, but I am *not* a physician. When you read this section, please remember that these are questions recently diagnosed prostate cancer patients and other presumably healthy men have asked me over the past two years and that the answers are mine based on my personal experiences. I was asked many other technical medical questions by this same group of men, and when asked I always told them to speak to a physician they trusted. I do not have the training to answer such technical questions. I employ the following rule of thumb: if I did not experience it firsthand and need to research an answer, then I *do not answer* the question.* I also strongly believe that it is important for every man to develop a relationship of trust with his physician. As a result I have left technical questions out of this section. If you have technical questions, please consult a physician you trust. If you haven't spoken to a physician about prostate cancer, please take the time to speak with him or her so that you understand this terrible disease and the ways we can beat it!

- During your ten years of monitoring, what were your prostate-specific antigen (PSA) levels and the results of your digital rectal examinations (DREs)?

* Where citations of websites are used in this document it is my intention to add a level of precision to topics.

I had thirteen PSA tests during this period. I did not receive the level for the first test in June 2000, but the test result was noted as normal (my internist noted normal as less than 4.5). Subsequent test scores were (in order of test from oldest to most recent) 3.3, 4.6, 3.3, 3.2, 3.7, 3.1, 3.2, 3.8, 4.2, 4.2, unknown, and my final prebiopsy result of 7.3. In each of these instances I also had a DRE, and the results were always normal. After my third test, when my PSA level was 4.6, and for all subsequent tests my urologist recommended that I have a biopsy, but each time I refused until my last test of 7.3. During this period my urologists were also testing my free PSA level as well as the velocity of my PSA. You should certainly speak to your urologist about free PSA and velocity tests. I think it is also worth noting that I was not exhibiting any of the symptoms of prostate cancer.

- Did you have any of the other symptoms of prostate cancer?

  No. I did not. The signs and symptoms of prostate cancer include the following:[7]

  - *Weak urinary stream.*
  - *Frequent and/or urgent urination, especially at night.*
  - *Difficulty starting or stopping the urinary stream.*
  - *Incomplete emptying of the bladder.*
  - *Painful, burning urination.*
  - *Blood in the urine or semen.*
  - *Painful ejaculation.*
  - *Pain or stiffness in the lower back, hips, or upper thighs.*

- Were the PSA tests, DREs, or biopsy painful?

The PSA test is a simple blood test, and although I have a hard time looking at my blood being drawn, the test itself is painless. The DRE is uncomfortable, and at first it was a little embarrassing, but once I learned that I had cancer my concern about my health lessened my embarrassment. I once mentioned to my internist as he performed my DRE that I hated this exam. His answer was "What do you think, I enjoy doing this exam?" The biopsy is a different story. It is uncomfortable and somewhat painful, but in my ranking of pain it was no worse than a root canal and certainly less painful than passing a kidney stone. I have spoken to some men who claim it was terribly painful, whereas one man mentioned that he was put to sleep by his urologist and did not feel a thing.

- How would you characterize your behavior during the ten years of PSA testing?

Although I could characterize my behavior as "watchful waiting," I think that would give me too much credit. It might better be characterized as "irrational waiting." You see, my waiting was based on ignorance, fear, and denial. From the beginning I knew very little about the prostate, its function, or prostate cancer for fear of learning too much. I never asked specific questions, and what little research I did do was to support my belief that I did not have cancer. I felt great and had no symptoms, hence my denial that there was any chance that I had cancer. This was just another form of Pat Walsh's "Don't ask don't tell" policy regarding my health: don't ask questions if the answer may scare you, and don't tell or talk to anyone about your concerns.

- Why did you choose to have minimally invasive robotic surgery over other options?

When I am asked why I chose a robotic prostatectomy my answer is simple: my urologist told me that is what I should do. I have spoken to other men who have researched various options and can cite the benefits and risks of each, but in my case I just followed my urologist's recommendation. I knew about robotic surgery and the benefits of minimally invasive surgery from my professional dealings in the field of cardiac surgery. After the biopsy showed that I had cancer and the pathology report showed a lot of cancer, denial was no longer an option. I trusted my urologist; he had successfully treated my father-in-law's bladder cancer and he had successfully gotten me to address my situation by employing a direct, caring, and forceful manner, so I went forward with his suggestion based on that trust.

- What criteria did you use to choose your surgeon?

I looked for the surgeons who were getting the best results and had performed the most surgeries. I asked whether the surgeons performed all of the surgeries themselves or if they were the teacher in the operating room, guiding others as they performed the surgery. If that had been the end of my selection process I trust that I would have found a surgeon who could have successfully treated my prostate cancer, but for me that was not enough! You have to find a surgeon you believe in! Trust that the surgeon can successfully perform the surgery is not enough. Believing and knowing that the surgeon and his team will be there for you and your family during the entire process, from presurgery to surgery to recovery, should be your goal. I cannot overemphasize this. You will need your surgeon and his team for so much, so make sure they have an infrastructure in place that will support your needs as you battle and recover from prostate cancer. I think a good way to find this out is to speak to patients who have been treated by the surgeon and his team.

- How long was your surgery?

  I entered the hospital around nine-thirty in the morning on the day of the surgery. Paperwork took approximately an hour and a half. My surgery was scheduled for noon and took approximately two hours. That was followed by six hours in recovery before I was taken to my room. I was up and walking around that night.

- How much pain did you experience after your surgery?

  I experienced very little pain after the surgery, and other than the pain medication I was given intravenously during surgery I took only over-the-counter pain medication during my hospital stay and my recovery at home.

- How long were you in the hospital after your surgery?

  As I mentioned, I entered the hospital at nine-thirty the morning of my surgery and left the hospital by two in the afternoon the next day, so a little more than twenty-eight hours.

- Did you have a lot of gas after your surgery?

  No, but I have spoken to men who experienced severe gas for days after their surgeries. I do not know why our experiences were so different. I know that in my case I had to pass gas before I could be released from the hospital, and this was not a problem. I believe the reason that to some degree we all had gas was because during the surgery the area where the surgery is performed is inflated by pumping gas into the body.

This improves both visibility for the surgeon and maneuverability of the surgical tools.

- How long did you have the Foley drainage catheter, and what was your experience with it?

  I had the catheter for seven days. The first day at home was the most difficult. In addition to getting used to moving around with the catheter, the drainage tube, and drainage bag, you are also responsible for maintaining the system. I hope that you will have someone to assist you with this; nothing is that difficult to do alone, but teamwork surely helps. The drainage bag has to be emptied, the exit site has to be cleaned to prevent infection, and the tubes need to be taped to the body for security.

- How long did it take for you to get back to work after surgery?

  I returned to work forty-seven days after my surgery, but I have spoken to men who have returned to work in a week after a robotic prostatectomy. I imagine some of the variables that impact how long you are out of work are the type of work you do (if your job includes the lifting of heavy objects I am sure this will affect when you can return), how well you heal, and whether you experience any complications. Based on my conversations with other men who had a robotic prostatectomy, my period away from work seems longer than most. I had complications that extended my time: first was an abscess that set me back approximately three weeks, including five days of hospitalization, and second was a kidney stone that I passed at the end of my recovery that resulted in a few days' delay in my return to work.

- How long did you have urinary leaking or dripping; what did you do about it?

I experienced some degree of urinary leaking during the entire period I was out of work; some of this was related to the abscess that developed around my bladder. Prior to the abscess I was making significant progress in controlling my urinary flow. I attribute this success to regularly doing my Kegel exercises and staying away from alcohol. The Kegel exercises strengthen the muscles in the pelvic area that you need to control urinary flow. Alcohol, on the other hand, tends to relax muscles, so until I had my muscles working again I stayed away from alcohol. The abscess worked against my urinary control by pushing down on the bladder and uncontrollably forcing the urine out of my bladder. Once the abscess cleared up, my control improved almost immediately. Dripping is an entirely different issue. I still experience some minor dripping when I lift heavy objects or when I unexpectedly sneeze. This does not occur very often, and I am not dripping a lot of fluid, so when it happens I try to focus on where I am in life as opposed to where I could have been if I had not had my cancer treated, and then I move forward!

- Is sex the same after the surgery?

My surgeon has a four-week rule: recovering patients are not allowed to have sex until four weeks after their surgery. When those four weeks passed, I immediately had sex and everything worked fine, with one significant difference: I had an erection and the sensations of ejaculation and climax, but there was no semen. My nerves were intact, but without a prostate or seminal vesicles, I was able to have sex without the mess. I have heard men characterize this as dry sex. I know this lack of semen would not be the ideal situation for a younger man who wanted to have children, but in my case, this is fine.

- Do you consider yourself cured of your prostate cancer?

  No, I am not cured, but I am a prostate cancer survivor and as a prostate cancer survivor I will have to have my blood tested on a regular basis for the rest of my life to monitor the level of PSA. After radical prostatectomy or radiation therapy, rising levels of PSA indicate residual disease or recurrence.[8] *This seems like a small price to pay for the wonderful life I lead!*

ABOUT THE AUTHOR

Pat is married and lives with his wife Isabel in Cranford and Stone Harbor, New Jersey; they have three grown children, a grandchild, and two golden retrievers. Pat was a successful businessman working in the medical device industry for the last twenty years.

Through the hard-hitting words of a concerned urologist, Pat took the necessary steps to end a decade-long denial and was diagnosed with prostate cancer in 2010 followed by a robotic prostatectomy in February 2011. His yearlong journey inspired him to share his experience and raise awareness for this potentially life-threatening disease.

Pat can be reached at: ptwadvisors@yahoo.com.

ENDNOTES

1 SEER Training Modules, Cancer Registration & Surveillance Modules specifically *Prostate Cancer*. US National Institutes of Health, National Cancer Institute. Access on 24 January 2014 http://www.training.seer.cancer.gov/prostate/intro/risk.html

2 SEER Training Modules, Cancer Registration & Surveillance Modules specifically *Prostate Cancer*. US National Institutes of Health, National Cancer Institute. Access on 24 January 2014 http://www.training.seer.cancer.gov/prostate/intro/symptoms.html

3 SEER Training Modules, Cancer Registration & Surveillance Modules specifically *Prostate Cancer*. US National Institutes of Health, National Cancer Institute. Access on 24 January 2014 http://www.training.seer.cancer.gov/prostate/intro/

4 SEER Training Modules, Cancer Registration & Surveillance Modules specifically *Prostate Cancer*. US National Institutes of Health, National Cancer Institute. Access on 24 January 2014 http://www.training.seer.cancer.gov/prostate/abstract-code-stage/extent/markers.html

5 PBS.org: Danger: UXB. Masterpiece Theatre Archive. Access confirmed on 8 January 2014 available at: http://www.pbs.org/wgbh/masterpiece/archive/55/55.html

6 SEER Training Modules, Cancer Registration & Surveillance Modules specifically *Prostate Cancer*. US National Institutes of Health, National Cancer Institute. Access on 24 January 2014 http://www.training.seer.cancer.gov/prostate/abstract-code-stage/extent/markers.html

7 SEER Training Modules, Cancer Registration & Surveillance Modules specifically *Prostate Cancer.* US National Institutes of Health, National Cancer Institute. Access on 24 January 2014 http://www.training.seer.cancer.gov/prostate/intro/symptoms.html

8 SEER Training Modules, Cancer Registration & Surveillance Modules specifically *Prostate Cancer.* US National Institutes of Health, National Cancer Institute. Access on 24 January 2014 http://www.training.seer.cancer.gov/prostate/abstract-code-stage/extent/markers.html

Made in the USA
Middletown, DE
01 July 2016